INSULIN RESISTANCE DIET BOOK GUIDE

The Role of Exercise in Insulin Sensitivity

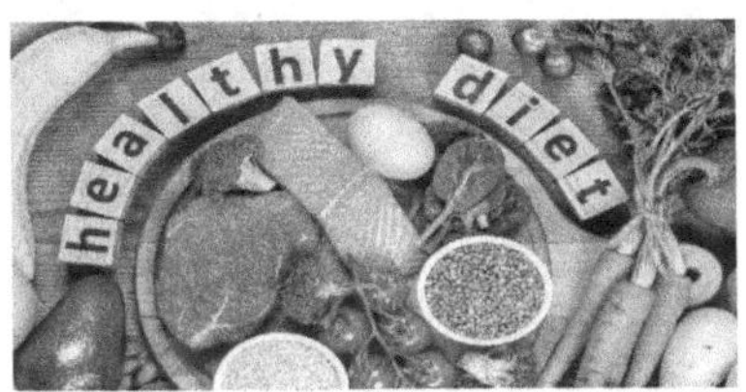

THERESA VIGUE

Table of Contents

This comprehensive table of contents will guide readers through, managing, and improving their insulin resistance through dietary and lifestyle changes.

Introduction

Understanding the Power of Food in Overcoming Insulin Resistance

In a world where dietary choices have a profound impact on our health, understanding the role of food in managing insulin resistance is a critical step towards reclaiming well-being. Welcome to the "Insulin Resistance Diet Guide," a comprehensive resource designed to shed light on the intricate relationship between what we eat and our body's response to insulin.

Insulin resistance, a condition where the body's cells struggle to respond to insulin's signals, has become a pervasive health concern. Its far-reaching implications extend beyond blood sugar control and touch on weight management, cardiovascular health, and even our risk of developing type 2 diabetes.

But there is hope.

The power to combat insulin resistance lies in our daily choices, particularly our dietary decisions. This book aims to unravel the complexities of this condition and equip you with the knowledge, tools, and strategies needed to make informed choices that can significantly improve your health.

Throughout the pages of this guide, we will embark on a journey of discovery, exploring the fundamental concepts of insulin resistance and how they relate to our dietary habits. You'll learn how your body processes food, why certain foods can either exacerbate or alleviate insulin resistance, and practical steps to craft a balanced, insulin-friendly diet.

We understand that embracing dietary changes can be challenging, but it's a journey well worth undertaking. The rewards include enhanced energy levels, improved blood sugar control, and a reduced risk of developing related health issues. This book is here to support and guide you every step of the way.

Whether you're grappling with insulin resistance or seeking proactive measures to prevent its onset, this book is your compass on the path to better health. It offers not only knowledge but also practical meal plans, delicious recipes, and lifestyle recommendations that will empower you to take control of your well-being.

Are you ready to transform your relationship with food and, in turn, your relationship with insulin? The journey begins here, with the insights and strategies within the pages of the "Insulin Resistance Diet Guide." It's time to embrace a healthier, more vibrant future. Let's embark on this transformative journey together.

Understanding Insulin Resistance

Insulin resistance is a complex metabolic condition that has gained significant attention in the realm of health and wellness. To comprehend this condition, it's essential to grasp the basic principles of insulin and how it functions in our bodies.

The Role of Insulin

Insulin is a hormone produced by the pancreas, and it plays a central role in regulating our blood sugar levels. When we consume carbohydrates, our digestive system breaks them down into glucose, a form of sugar. This glucose is then released into the bloodstream, causing a rise in blood sugar levels.

In response to elevated blood sugar, the pancreas releases insulin. Insulin acts as a key that unlocks our cells, allowing them to take in glucose from the bloodstream. This serves two critical purposes:

Energy Utilization: Cells use glucose for energy. It's the fuel that keeps our bodies functioning optimally.

Blood Sugar Regulation: By allowing cells to take in glucose, insulin helps lower blood sugar levels back to a stable range.

In individuals with normal insulin sensitivity, this process works seamlessly. However, in cases of insulin resistance, something goes awry.

Understanding Insulin Resistance

Insulin resistance occurs when the body's cells become less responsive to insulin signals. It's as if the key (insulin) can't unlock the door (cell) as effectively as it should. As a result, several critical issues arise:

Elevated Blood Sugar: With cells resistant to insulin, glucose remains in the bloodstream for longer periods, leading to elevated blood sugar levels, a condition known as hyperglycemia.

Pancreatic Overcompensation: The pancreas attempts to compensate for insulin resistance by producing even more insulin. This can lead to higher levels of insulin in the blood, a condition called hyperinsulinemia.

Increased Fat Storage: Insulin is also involved in regulating fat storage. When insulin is abundant, the body is more prone to storing excess calories as fat, contributing to weight gain and obesity.

Risk of Type 2 Diabetes: Prolonged insulin resistance can eventually lead to the development of type 2 diabetes, a chronic condition characterized by persistently high blood sugar levels.

Understanding insulin resistance is the first step towards managing and mitigating its impact on your health. In the following chapters, we'll delve deeper into the causes, risk factors, and potential health implications of insulin resistance, empowering you to take proactive steps toward a healthier future.

Why Your Diet Matters

- In the grand tapestry of life, what we eat and how we eat it plays a pivotal role. Our dietary choices extend far beyond mere sustenance; they hold the power to shape our health, impact our well-being, and influence our susceptibility to a range of health conditions. One of the most significant conditions affected by our diet is insulin resistance, and understanding why your diet matters in the context of this condition is paramount.
- The Food-Insulin Connection
- The food we consume directly influences our blood sugar levels and, by extension, our insulin response. Certain foods cause rapid spikes in blood sugar, while others provide slow and steady energy release. The choice between these types of foods is a defining factor in whether your diet supports or hinders insulin sensitivity.
- Carbohydrates: Carbohydrates are a primary source of glucose in our diets. The type of carbohydrates you consume matters greatly. Simple carbohydrates, like sugar and refined grains, cause

rapid and sharp increases in blood sugar
levels, while complex carbohydrates,
such as whole grains and legumes, lead
to more gradual and controlled
increases.

- Fibrer: Foods rich in fibre, such as
  vegetables, fruits, and whole grains,
  slow down the absorption of glucose,
  helping to maintain stable blood sugar
  levels. This not only benefits insulin
  sensitivity but also supports feelings of
  fullness and weight management.
- Proteins and Fats: Including adequate
  protein and healthy fats in your diet can
  help balance your meals and prevent
  blood sugar spikes. Protein and fats
  contribute to satiety, reducing the urge
  to overindulge in high-sugar, high-carb
  foods.
- Weight and Insulin Resistance
- Beyond blood sugar control, your diet
  plays a pivotal role in weight
  management. Excess body weight,
  particularly visceral fat (fat around the
  abdomen), is strongly associated with
  insulin resistance. Unhealthy eating
  patterns can lead to weight gain,
  exacerbating insulin resistance and

increasing the risk of related health issues.

- The Inflammatory Factor
- Dietary choices can also impact inflammation in the body. Chronic inflammation is a contributing factor to insulin resistance and several chronic diseases. Foods high in added sugars and unhealthy fats can promote inflammation, while an anti-inflammatory diet, rich in fruits, vegetables, and omega-3 fatty acids, can help reduce inflammation and improve insulin sensitivity.
- In this "Insulin Resistance Diet Guide," we'll explore the specific dietary principles and strategies that can help you manage and even reverse insulin resistance. Whether you're seeking to prevent the condition, manage your blood sugar levels, or enhance your overall health, your diet is a powerful tool that can be harnessed for a brighter, healthier future.
- As we journey through the following chapters, you'll gain insights into the principles of the insulin resistance diet, foods to include and avoid, meal planning strategies, and more. It's time

to take control of your dietary choices
and harness the transformative potential
of your meals in the battle against
insulin resistance.

The Insulin Resistance Connection

Insulin resistance is a metabolic puzzle with profound implications for your health. To unlock this puzzle, it's essential to understand the intricate relationship between insulin, and blood sugar, and how insulin resistance fits into the picture.

The Role of Insulin

Insulin, often referred to as the body's "gatekeeper," is a hormone produced by the pancreas. Its primary role is to regulate blood sugar (glucose) levels in your body. Here's how it works:

Glucose Regulation: When you consume carbohydrates, your digestive system breaks them down into glucose, a form of sugar. This glucose enters your bloodstream, causing blood sugar levels to rise.

Insulin Release: In response to elevated blood sugar, the pancreas releases insulin into the bloodstream. Think of insulin as a key that unlocks the doors of your body's cells, allowing glucose to enter.

Energy Utilization: Inside your cells, glucose is used for energy. It powers your muscles, brain, and all other bodily functions.

Blood Sugar Control: As glucose enters the cells, blood sugar levels return to a stable range. This is vital for your health, as consistently high blood sugar can lead to various complications.

What Happens in Insulin Resistance?

In individuals with insulin resistance, a glitch occurs in this finely-tuned process. Your cells become less responsive to the signals of insulin, which leads to several critical consequences:

Elevated Blood Sugar: With cells resisting insulin's attempts to let glucose in, blood sugar remains high. This condition is called hyperglycemia.

Pancreatic Overcompensation: To counteract the resistance, your pancreas releases even more insulin. This can result in elevated levels of insulin in your bloodstream, a condition known as hyperinsulinemia.

Increased Fat Storage: Insulin is also involved in regulating fat storage. When insulin is abundant, the body is more likely to store excess calories as fat, contributing to weight gain and obesity.

Risk of Type 2 Diabetes: Prolonged insulin resistance can ultimately lead to the development of type 2 diabetes, a chronic condition characterized by persistently high blood sugar levels.

Understanding the Complexity

The development of insulin resistance is influenced by a myriad of factors, including genetics, lifestyle choices, and overall health. While genetics may play a role, lifestyle choices such as diet and physical activity have a significant impact on the onset and progression of insulin resistance.

In the following sections of this guide, we will delve deeper into the causes, risk factors, and potential health implications of insulin resistance. Armed with this knowledge, you'll be better prepared to navigate the complexities of insulin resistance and, more importantly, to take proactive steps toward managing and improving your health.

Insulin resistance is a metabolic condition that lies at the intersection of biology, genetics, and lifestyle choices. To comprehend the basics of insulin resistance, it's crucial to explore what it is, how it develops, and the impact it has on your health.

What Is Insulin Resistance?

Insulin resistance is a condition in which the body's cells, primarily those in muscles, fat, and the liver, become less responsive to the effects of insulin. As a result, the normal processes of glucose uptake and utilization are impaired. To visualize this, think of insulin as a key that unlocks the doors of your cells to allow glucose (sugar) to enter. When you have insulin resistance, these cellular doors don't open as easily, making it more challenging for glucose to enter your cells.

How Does Insulin Resistance Develop?

The development of insulin resistance is a complex interplay of genetic, environmental, and lifestyle factors. Several key elements contribute to its onset.

Genetics: Some individuals may be genetically predisposed to insulin resistance, meaning they have a higher likelihood of developing the condition due to their family history.

Obesity: Excess body fat, particularly abdominal fat, is strongly associated with insulin resistance. The fat cells release substances that can interfere with insulin signaling.

Physical Inactivity: A sedentary lifestyle can contribute to weight gain and worsen insulin resistance. Regular physical activity helps improve insulin sensitivity.

Poor Diet: Diets high in sugar, refined carbohydrates, and saturated fats can promote weight gain and inflammation, both of which can worsen insulin resistance.

Chronic Inflammation: Inflammatory processes in the body can interfere with insulin signaling, making cells less responsive to insulin.

Hormonal Imbalances: Conditions like polycystic ovary syndrome (PCOS) and hormonal disorders can increase the risk of insulin resistance.

Health Implications of Insulin Resistance

Insulin resistance is more than just a metabolic hiccup. It's associated with a range of health complications and risks, including:

Type 2 Diabetes: Prolonged insulin resistance can lead to the development of type 2 diabetes, a chronic condition characterized by elevated blood sugar levels.

Cardiovascular Issues: Insulin resistance is closely linked to heart disease and an increased risk of high blood pressure, high cholesterol, and atherosclerosis.

Metabolic Syndrome: People with insulin resistance are often diagnosed with metabolic syndrome, a cluster of conditions that increase the risk of heart disease, stroke, and type 2 diabetes.

Fatty Liver Disease: Insulin resistance can contribute to the accumulation of fat in the liver, leading to non-alcoholic fatty liver disease (NAFLD).

Weight Management Challenges: Insulin resistance can make it more difficult to lose weight and maintain a healthy weight.

Understanding the basics of insulin resistance is the first step toward managing and mitigating its impact on your health. In the following chapters of this guide, we'll delve deeper into the causes, risk factors, and strategies for addressing insulin resistance, empowering you to take control of your well-being   Causes and Risk Factors

Insulin resistance is a complex metabolic condition influenced by a combination of genetic and lifestyle factors. While its exact causes can vary from person to person, certain common factors and risk elements are known to contribute to the development of insulin resistance:

Genetics

Family History: A family history of insulin resistance or type 2 diabetes can increase an individual's risk. Genetic factors play a significant role in determining susceptibility.

Obesity

Excess Body Fat: Obesity, especially when it involves the accumulation of visceral fat (fat around the abdominal organs), is a major risk factor. Fat cells release substances that can interfere with insulin signaling.

Physical Inactivity

Sedentary Lifestyle: A lack of physical activity can lead to weight gain and worsen insulin resistance. Exercise helps improve insulin sensitivity.

Diet

High Sugar and Refined Carbohydrate Intake: Diets high in added sugars and refined carbohydrates can lead to rapid blood sugar spikes and weight gain, contributing to insulin resistance.

High Saturated and Trans Fat Intake: A diet rich in unhealthy fats, especially saturated and trans fats, can promote inflammation and insulin resistance.

Chronic Inflammation

Inflammatory Conditions: Chronic inflammation in the body can interfere with insulin signaling, making cells less responsive to insulin.

Hormonal Factors

Polycystic Ovary Syndrome (PCOS): PCOS is a common hormonal disorder in women that is often associated with insulin resistance.

Hormonal Imbalances: Certain hormonal imbalances can increase the risk of insulin resistance.

Age

Age-Related Changes: Insulin sensitivity tends to decrease with age, making older

individuals more susceptible to insulin
resistance.

Medications

Certain Medications: Some medications,
such as certain antipsychotics,
corticosteroids, and antiretroviral drugs,
can contribute to insulin resistance.

Sleep Disorders

Sleep Apnea: Sleep apnea, a condition
characterized by interrupted breathing
during sleep, has been linked to insulin
resistance.

Stress

Chronic Stress: Prolonged exposure to
high levels of stress can affect hormones
that regulate blood sugar and contribute
to insulin resistance.

Smoking

Tobacco Use: Smoking is associated with insulin resistance and an increased risk of type 2 diabetes.

Understanding these causes and risk factors is essential for both preventing and managing insulin resistance. While some factors, like genetics, can't be changed, many lifestyle-related risk factors can be addressed through dietary improvements, regular physical activity, stress management, and other health-conscious choices. By taking proactive steps to mitigate these risks, individuals can reduce their chances of developing insulin resistance and its associated health complications

Insulin resistance is more than just a metabolic anomaly; it has far-reaching implications for your health. When left unmanaged, insulin resistance can contribute to a range of health complications and increase the risk of chronic diseases. Here are some of the key health implications of insulin resistance:

Type 2 Diabetes

Perhaps the most well-known consequence, prolonged insulin resistance can lead to the development of type 2 diabetes. In this condition, the body cannot effectively use insulin to regulate blood sugar, resulting in chronically elevated blood sugar levels.

Cardiovascular Issues

Insulin resistance is closely linked to heart disease and an increased risk of cardiovascular problems, including:

High Blood Pressure (Hypertension): Insulin resistance can contribute to high blood pressure, which is a major risk factor for heart disease.

High Cholesterol Levels: People with insulin resistance often have unhealthy cholesterol profiles, with elevated levels of LDL (bad) cholesterol and lower levels of HDL (good) cholesterol.

Atherosclerosis: Insulin resistance is associated with the development of fatty deposits in the arteries, which can narrow and harden the blood vessels (atherosclerosis).

Metabolic Syndrome

Insulin resistance is a central feature of metabolic syndrome, a cluster of conditions that increase the risk of heart disease, stroke, and type 2 diabetes. Metabolic syndrome includes symptoms such as abdominal obesity, high blood pressure, high blood sugar, and abnormal cholesterol levels.

Fatty Liver Disease

Insulin resistance can contribute to the accumulation of fat in the liver, leading to non-alcoholic fatty liver disease (NAFLD). In severe cases, NAFLD can progress to non-alcoholic steatohepatitis (NASH), which is associated with inflammation and liver damage.

Weight Management Challenges

Insulin resistance can make it more difficult to lose weight and maintain a healthy weight. It promotes fat storage, particularly in the abdominal area, and reduces the body's ability to burn stored fat for energy.

Increased Risk of Stroke

People with insulin resistance have a higher risk of stroke, which is often related to the impact of insulin resistance on the cardiovascular system.

Kidney Disease

Insulin resistance may contribute to the development and progression of kidney disease, particularly in individuals with diabetes.

Reproductive Health Issues

In women, insulin resistance is associated with polycystic ovary syndrome (PCOS), a hormonal disorder that can lead to irregular menstrual cycles, fertility problems, and other reproductive health issues.

Inflammation

Chronic inflammation is a common feature of insulin resistance and can contribute to various health issues, including autoimmune diseases and certain types of cancer.

Understanding the potential health implications of insulin resistance underscores the importance of proactive management and prevention. Making lifestyle changes such as adopting a healthy diet, engaging in regular physical activity, and managing stress can go a long way in mitigating the risks associated with insulin resistance and improving overall health and well-being.

Best thing for insulin

insulin is an important hormone for regulating the movement of nutrients into and out of your cells if your cells resist its effects insulin cannot do its job creating inflammation and making it hard to lose weight insulin resistance is a common condition but you can do things to make yourselves more sensitive instead of just telling you to sleep better eat better and move better this video will share practical things you can start doing today to reduce insulin resistance and the best thing is it won't cost you a dime you may have come to this video because you were told that you had insulin resistance pre-diabetes metabolic syndrome or you have trouble losing weight and suspect that insulin resistance may be a root cause this video will show you how to reduce the condition if you need some background information i will point you to two of my previous videos the first provides a four minute explanation of insulin resistance the second shares the signs to look for the first was filmed way back in 2016 when i was still trying to figure out if there was anything to this whole youtube thing so the information is good but the video quality shows that we've come a long way since then anyway we know that insulin resistance increases with increasing fat mass especially when there is a lot of visceral or belly fat that's because visceral fat is more metabolically active than subcutaneous fat that you can pinch under your skin as a result belly fat releases more free fatty acids into the bloodstream promoting insulin resistance so of the strategies for reducing this condition improving your diet will have the biggest payoff and that involves changing your food choices not just the amount you eat when your body is insulin resistant blood insulin levels run high which is a state that encourages fat storage therefore if you are insulin resistant just eating less of the same foods will lead to frustration because that internal fat storing state is still in place to work toward insulin sensitivity you want to focus your food choices on those that naturally keep your blood sugar low because less sugar in the blood means less insulin is needed carbohydrates cause blood sugar levels to rise the most and fats cause the least impact therefore low carb high fat diets like the keto diet naturally stabilize blood sugar which is an effect that has been shown to improve insulin sensitivity not all carbs however are created equal a cupcake and romaine lettuce are both classified as carbohydrates however only the

cupcake will spike your blood sugar so while
you want to go low carb to reduce insulin
resistance you do not need to go no carb also
not all fats are created equal for instance
mass-produced vegetable and seed oils like
soybean oil create inflammation in the body
worsening insulin resistance healthy fats are a
hallmark of the mediterranean diet and as with
low carb diets the mediterranean diet has been
shown to improve insulin sensitivity when you
marry these two eating styles you give insulin
resistance a one-two punch because you reduce
inflammation and lose weight with a
mediterranean-style keto diet your main source
of calories come from fish and seafood
low-carb vegetables and extra virgin oils
poultry and eggs provide additional sources of
protein meat cheese yogurt nuts seeds and
low-carb fruits are also a part of the diet in
moderation to follow a mediterranean keto diet
think salad for lunch and lean protein with
cooked vegetables for dinner you can start
eating this way tonight i put recipes for my
low-carb high-fat salad baked salmon with dill
sauce and garlic green beans with pine nuts in
a blog post that goes with this video you can
download them for free by going to
drbeckyfitness.com forward slash reduce
insulin resistance and i will add that if you find

that you enjoy eating this way i also have a cookbook with more than 45 mediterranean keto recipes organized into two weekly meal plans available on my website as for breakfast you have options including eggs full fat yogurt or skipping it to utilize intermittent fasting intermittent fasting is a valuable and easy to implement tool in your strategy to reduce insulin resistance during your fasting hours when there's no food coming in there's no rise in blood sugar or insulin making your body more insulin sensitive over time and reducing your risk of obesity and diabetes intermittent fasting will meet you where you are at if you have never fasted before i encourage you to start with an overnight fast of 12 hours and work up to a 16 8 fast meaning that you fast for 16 hours and consume calories during an eight hour eating window for instance you can skip breakfast have lunch at 11am and finish dinner by 7pm and you don't have to skip breakfast to perform intermittent fasting in fact once you are comfortable with 16 8 fasting consider moving your eating window to earlier in the day for instance start eating by 7am and finish eating for the day by 3 p.m this form of fasting referred to as early time restricted eating has been shown to improve insulin sensitivity and improve the function of the pancreas which is the organ that produces insulin getting regular exercise makes it easier for your cells to take in glucose essentially reversing the resistance they once had what type of exercise is best well as it turns out the best one is the one that you are willing to do it has been found that all forms of exercise help so whether you enjoy aerobic style exercises like walking or riding a bike or prefer lifting weights at the gym you will benefit improvements in the way you eat and exercise will improve insulin sensitivity you can further your progress with better sleep and stress control these two pieces of advice are often handed out but rarely linked to a practical tool that makes a difference i have found that an overactive mind ramps up stress and makes it hard to sleep there are apps out there geared toward calming your thoughts one that i've found useful is libby the nice thing is that it is free because it's an app that allows you to download audio books from your local library all you need is a library card which you can get online simply find libby in the app store of your phone attach your library card number and search for audiobooks i will list a few of the books i've enjoyed in the video description in my opinion the distraction of a good book is a thing from our past that we need to revive the app also has a sleep timer so your story automatically pauses as you fall asleep here's what your plan for reducing insulin resistance looks like you'll start by focusing your food choices on foods that stabilize your blood sugar this can be accomplished by eating a salad topped with healthy fats for lunch and fish with cooked vegetables for dinner for free recipes or my mediterranean keto cookbook see the links in the description area below this video to further improve insulin sensitivity eat within a shortened eating window working up to an early time restricted eating pattern where you finish eating for the day by 3 p.m make a concerted effort to move more as any form of exercise helps your cells take in glucose also let technology help you control stress and improve sleep utilize the free libby app and decompress with a good audio book you'll find links to all the materials in the video description below this video thanks for watching please share this video with your community and join my community by clicking the subscribe button have a great rest of your day.

The Role of Insulin

Insulin is a remarkable hormone with a pivotal role in regulating blood sugar (glucose) levels in the body. To appreciate the importance of insulin and how it operates, it's essential to understand its multifaceted functions:

Glucose Uptake: The primary function of insulin is to facilitate the uptake of glucose by cells. When you eat carbohydrates, they are broken down into glucose, which enters the bloodstream. In response to elevated blood sugar, the pancreas secretes insulin. This hormone acts as a key that unlocks the doors of your cells, allowing glucose to enter. It's within the cells that glucose is converted into energy.

Blood Sugar Control: The actions of insulin helps regulate blood sugar levels, ensuring that they remain within a narrow and stable range. This balance is vital for the body's overall health and functionality. Chronically high blood sugar levels can lead to various complications, including damage to blood vessels, nerves, and organs.

Storage of Excess Glucose: When there is an excess of glucose in the bloodstream, typically after a meal, insulin encourages the storage of this surplus glucose in the liver and muscles as glycogen. Glycogen serves as a short-term energy reserve. Once the glycogen stores are filled, any extra glucose is converted into fat and stored for long-term energy needs.

Protein Synthesis: Insulin also plays a role in the synthesis of proteins. It helps cells take in amino acids, which are the building blocks of proteins. This is essential for cell repair and growth.

Inhibition of Fat Breakdown: Insulin has an inhibitory effect on the breakdown of fat (lipolysis). When insulin is abundant, it signals to the body that glucose is available for energy, and this reduces the breakdown of fat for energy.

Regulation of Metabolism: Beyond its effects on glucose, insulin influences the metabolism of various nutrients, including carbohydrates, fats, and proteins. It promotes the storage of nutrients during periods of abundance and their release during times of need.

Cell Growth and Differentiation: Insulin is also involved in the growth and differentiation of cells, which is important for tissue development and repair.

In summary, insulin is a key player in the body's intricate dance of maintaining stable blood sugar levels and efficiently utilizing energy sources. It helps regulate glucose uptake by cells, store excess glucose, and manage various aspects of metabolism. The absence or dysfunction of insulin, as seen in type 1 diabetes, can lead to uncontrolled high blood sugar and its associated health issues, highlighting the critical role that insulin plays in our well-being.

How Insulin Works

Insulin is a hormone produced by the pancreas with a crucial role in regulating blood sugar (glucose) levels in the body. To understand how insulin works, let's delve into the intricate process that occurs when you eat and how insulin orchestrates glucose management.

Digestion and Glucose Release

When you eat, the food is broken down in your digestive system. Carbohydrates, such as starches and sugars, are converted into glucose, which is released into your bloodstream.

Blood Sugar Elevation

As glucose enters your bloodstream, your blood sugar levels rise. This increase in blood sugar acts as a signal that your cells need energy.

Insulin Secretion

In response to elevated blood sugar, the pancreas, a gland located behind your stomach, releases insulin into your bloodstream.

Unlocking Cellular Doors

Insulin is like a key that fits into receptors on the surface of your body's cells, particularly muscle, fat, and liver cells. When insulin binds to these receptors, it triggers a series of cellular events.

Glucose Entry into Cells

The key function of insulin is to enable the uptake of glucose by your cells. Once the cell receptors receive the signal from insulin, they open up to allow glucose to enter.

Energy Production

Inside the cells, glucose is converted into energy through a process called cellular respiration. This energy is used to fuel various bodily functions, including muscle contraction, brain activity, and maintaining body temperature.

Blood Sugar Reduction

As glucose enters the cells and is utilized for energy, the amount of glucose in your bloodstream decreases. This leads to a reduction in blood sugar levels.

Storage of Excess Glucose

If there is more glucose in your bloodstream than your cells need for immediate energy, insulin encourages the storage of this surplus glucose. It first fills up the glycogen stores in the liver and muscles. Any remaining excess glucose is converted into fat and stored for future energy needs.

Blood Sugar Balance

The actions of insulin help maintain blood sugar levels within a narrow and stable range, preventing them from becoming too high or too low.

Feedback Mechanism

The body continuously monitors blood sugar levels, and when they drop too low, another hormone called glucagon is released by the pancreas to raise blood sugar levels. Insulin and glucagon work together to keep blood sugar levels in balance.

In summary, insulin is the body's key player in regulating blood sugar and managing the utilization and storage of glucose. It ensures that glucose is delivered to the cells for energy, stored when there's an excess, and maintains blood sugar levels within a healthy range. When this finely tuned system is disrupted, as in the case of insulin resistance, it can lead to problems with blood sugar control and various health complications.

Insulin and Blood Sugar

The relationship between insulin and blood sugar is a fundamental aspect of our body's metabolism. Insulin plays a critical role in maintaining blood sugar levels within a narrow and healthy range. Here's how the interaction between insulin and blood sugar works:

Blood Sugar Regulation

After you eat, especially when your meal contains carbohydrates, your digestive system breaks down the food into glucose, a type of sugar. Glucose enters your bloodstream and causes your blood sugar levels to rise.

Insulin Secretion

In response to the increase in blood sugar, the pancreas, a gland located behind your stomach, releases insulin into your bloodstream. This is like an

automatic response to the rise in blood
sugar levels.

Unlocking Cellular Doors

Insulin acts as a key that fits into
receptors on the surface of your body's
cells, particularly muscle, fat, and liver
cells. When insulin binds to these
receptors, it sends a signal to the cells.

Glucose Uptake

Once the cell receptors receive the signal
from insulin, they open up and allow
glucose to enter. This process is crucial
because it ensures that glucose is taken
out of the bloodstream and into the cells
where it can be used for energy.

Blood Sugar Reduction

As glucose is taken up by the cells and
utilized for energy, the amount of
glucose in your bloodstream decreases.
This leads to a reduction in blood sugar

levels, bringing them back to a stable range.

Maintaining Balance

The actions of insulin, along with other factors like glucagon (a hormone that raises blood sugar levels when they drop too low), work together to keep blood sugar levels in balance. The goal is to prevent blood sugar from becoming too high (hyperglycemia) or too low (hypoglycemia).

Insulin is a key player in this delicate balancing act, helping to keep blood sugar levels stable and ensuring that glucose is available for your body's energy needs. When insulin isn't working effectively, as in the case of insulin resistance, it can lead to issues with blood sugar control, potentially resulting in elevated blood sugar levels, a condition known as hyperglycemia. This is a hallmark feature of type 2 diabetes, a condition that often involves insulin resistance and requires careful

management to avoid the complications
associated with high blood sugar.

While insulin is primarily known for its role in regulating blood sugar and glucose utilization, it also plays a significant role in the storage and metabolism of fats. The relationship between insulin and fat storage is essential for understanding how the hormone affects weight and body composition. Here's how it works:

Glucose Uptake

When you consume carbohydrates, they are broken down into glucose, which enters your bloodstream. Elevated blood sugar levels signal the need for insulin to regulate them.

Insulin Secretion

The pancreas releases insulin in response to increased blood sugar levels. Insulin's primary function is to facilitate

the uptake of glucose by cells, enabling
them to use it for energy.

Storage of Excess Glucose

If there is more glucose in your
bloodstream than your cells require for
immediate energy needs, insulin
encourages the storage of this surplus
glucose.

The first step is filling up the glycogen
stores in the liver and muscles. Glycogen
is a form of stored glucose that can be
used when the body requires a quick
energy boost.

Conversion of Excess Glucose to Fat

If glycogen stores are already full,
insulin triggers the conversion of the
excess glucose into fat. This process is
known as lipogenesis. The fat is then
stored in fat cells (adipocytes)

throughout the body, particularly in adipose tissue, as triglycerides.

Fat Storage and Weight Gain

Insulin promotes the storage of fat and inhibits the breakdown of fat (lipolysis). When insulin levels are high, the body is more likely to store excess calories as fat.

Fat Utilization

When insulin levels are low, typically between meals or during periods of physical activity, the body can use stored fat for energy. This process involves the release of fatty acids from fat cells and their utilization by cells for energy.

Role in Weight Management

The relationship between insulin and fat storage has important implications for weight management. Elevated insulin levels, often resulting from a diet high in refined carbohydrates and sugars, can promote fat storage and make it more challenging to lose weight.

Understanding how insulin influences fat storage is key to making informed dietary choices. A diet that consistently leads to high insulin levels may contribute to weight gain and obesity. In contrast, a diet that supports healthy insulin levels, along with physical activity, can help manage weight and promote a healthier body composition. This is why many dietary

strategies for weight
management focus on
managing blood sugar
and insulin levels.

Understanding your level of insulin resistance is a crucial step in managing your health and making informed decisions about your lifestyle and dietary choices. This section will guide you through several methods to assess your insulin xvh 4 g . Keep in mind that these b can provide valuable insights, but for a comprehensive evaluation and personalized advice, it's essential to consult with a healthcare professional. Here are some approaches to assess your insulin :

Fasting Blood Sugar Test

This simple blood test measures your blood sugar levels after an overnight fast. Elevated fasting blood sugar levels may be an indicator of insulin resistance.

Hemoglobin A1c Test

The hemoglobin A1c test provides an estimate of your average blood sugar levels over the past two to three months. It's a reliable indicator of long-term blood sugar control.

Oral Glucose Tolerance Test (OGTT)

During this test, you'll drink a sugary solution, and your blood sugar levels will be monitored over a while. It can reveal how effectively your body processes glucose and responds to insulin.

Insulin Test

A fasting insulin test measures the level of insulin in your blood while you are fasting. Elevated insulin levels can indicate insulin resistance.

Home Glucose Monitoring

You can also monitor your blood sugar levels at home using a glucose meter. Regular tracking of your blood sugar levels can provide valuable information about your daily fluctuations.

Assess Your Factors

Consider your risk factors for insulin resistance. Factors such as family history, obesity, a sedentary lifestyle, and an unhealthy diet can increase your risk.

Body Measurements

Your waist circumference can be a practical indicator of insulin resistance. Abdominal obesity is strongly associated with insulin resistance.

Health Symptoms

Pay attention to common symptoms of insulin resistance, such as increased thirst, frequent urination, fatigue, and skin changes. These symptoms may prompt further evaluation.

Remember that no single test provides a complete picture of your insulin resistance. Combining multiple assessments and discussing the results with a healthcare professional is the most effective way to evaluate your insulin sensitivity accurately.

Once you have a better understanding of your insulin resistance status, you can tailor your lifestyle, diet, and potential medical interventions to better manage and improve your insulin sensitivity. The next section of this guide will explore strategies for managing and mitigating insulin resistance.

Recognizing the Signs of Insulin Resistance

Insulin resistance often develops gradually, and its symptoms can be subtle. It's essential to recognize the signs early to take proactive steps toward better health. While not everyone with insulin resistance will experience all of these signs, here are common indicators to be aware of:

Elevated Blood Sugar

One of the hallmark signs of insulin resistance is consistently elevated blood sugar levels, especially after meals. This can be identified through blood sugar testing, including fasting blood sugar and hemoglobin A1c tests.

Increased Hunger and Food Cravings

Insulin resistance can lead to hunger and cravings, particularly for sugary and high-carb foods. You may find it challenging to control your appetite.

Frequent Urination

Insulin resistance can lead to increased thirst and frequent urination, especially during the night.

Fatigue

Feeling tired, even after a full night's sleep, can be a common symptom. Insulin resistance may disrupt your energy metabolism.

Abdominal Obesity

Excess weight around the abdominal area is a significant risk factor for insulin resistance. Measuring your waist circumference can provide insights into this.

Skin Changes

Dark patches of skin on the neck, armpits, or other areas (acanthosis nigricans) can be a sign of insulin resistance.

Polycystic Ovary Syndrome (PCOS)

Women with insulin resistance may experience irregular menstrual cycles, fertility issues, and other symptoms of PCOS.

High Blood Pressure

Hypertension is commonly associated with insulin resistance and can increase the risk of cardiovascular problems.

High Cholesterol Levels

Elevated levels of triglycerides and LDL (bad) cholesterol and lower levels of HDL (good) cholesterol may be present in individuals with insulin resistance.

The presence of skin tags, which are small, soft growths on the skin, can sometimes be associated with insulin resistance.

Cognitive Issues

Some people with insulin resistance report difficulty concentrating and memory problems, often referred to as "brain fog."

Sleep Problems

Sleep disturbances, including sleep apnea, can be more common in individuals with insulin resistance.

Slow Wound Healing

Insulin resistance can slow down the body's ability to heal wounds and injuries.

It's important to note that not everyone with insulin resistance will exhibit all of these signs, and some individuals may experience symptoms more intensely than others. If you suspect insulin resistance or are experiencing these symptoms, it's advisable to consult with a healthcare professional for a thorough evaluation and appropriate guidance. Early recognition and management of insulin resistance can help reduce the risk of associated health complications and improve overall well-being.

Insulin resistance and the resulting increase in blood sugar levels can manifest in various symptoms. Common symptoms and signs associated with insulin resistance include:

Frequent Hunger: You may find yourself feeling hungry shortly after eating a meal.

Cravings for Sugary Foods: A strong desire for sugary or high-carbohydrate foods is a common symptom.

Increased Thirst: Insulin resistance can lead to increased thirst, and you may find yourself drinking more fluids than usual.

Frequent Urination: You might notice that you need to urinate more frequently, especially at night.

Fatigue: Feeling tired and lacking energy, even after a good night's sleep, is a common complaint.

Abdominal Weight Gain: Excess fat accumulation around the abdominal area, often referred to as an "apple-shaped" body, is associated with insulin resistance.

Dark Skin Patches: A condition called acanthosis nigricans can cause dark, velvety patches of skin, typically on the neck, armpits, or groin.

Polycystic Ovary Syndrome (PCOS): In women, insulin resistance is often linked to PCOS, which can cause irregular menstrual cycles, fertility issues, and other symptoms.

High Blood Pressure: Hypertension is commonly associated with insulin resistance and increases the risk of cardiovascular problems.

High Cholesterol: Elevated levels of triglycerides and LDL (bad) cholesterol, along with lower levels of HDL (good) cholesterol, may be present.

Skin Tags: Small, soft growths on the skin, known as skin tags, can sometimes be associated with insulin resistance.

Cognitive Issues: Difficulty concentrating, memory problems, and "brain fog" are symptoms some individuals with insulin resistance experience.

Sleep Disturbances: Sleep problems, including sleep apnea, can be more common in those with insulin resistance.

Slow Wound Healing: Wounds and injuries may take longer to heal in individuals with insulin resistance.

It's important to note that not everyone with insulin resistance will exhibit all of these symptoms, and the severity of symptoms can vary from person to person. If you suspect insulin resistance or are experiencing these symptoms, it's advisable to seek medical evaluation and guidance from a healthcare professional. Early recognition and management of insulin resistance can help reduce the risk of associated health complications and improve overall well-being.

Diagnostic Tests

Diagnosing insulin resistance typically involves a combination of clinical assessments, blood tests, and other measurements. Healthcare professionals use these tests and evaluations to determine the presence and severity of insulin resistance. Here are some diagnostic tests commonly used.

Fasting Blood Sugar Test (FBS): This test measures your blood sugar level after an overnight fast. Elevated fasting blood sugar levels may indicate insulin resistance.

Hemoglobin A1c (HbA1c) Test: The HbA1c test provides an estimate of your average blood sugar levels over the past two to three months. It's a reliable indicator of long-term blood sugar control.

Oral Glucose Tolerance Test (OGTT): During this test, you consume a sugary solution, and your blood sugar levels are monitored over some time. It can reveal how effectively your body processes glucose and responds to insulin.

Insulin Test: A fasting insulin test measures the level of insulin in your blood while you are fasting. Elevated insulin levels can indicate insulin resistance.

Home Glucose Monitoring: You can monitor your blood sugar levels at home using a glucose meter. Regular tracking of your blood sugar levels can provide valuable information about your daily fluctuations.

Body Measurements: Assessing waist circumference can provide insights into abdominal obesity, a strong risk factor for insulin resistance.

Clinical Evaluation: Your healthcare provider may perform a physical examination to check for symptoms or signs associated with insulin resistance, such as skin changes, acanthosis nigricans, or skin tags.

Risk Assessment: Your healthcare provider will consider your risk factors, including family history, obesity, sedentary lifestyle, and dietary habits.

Review of Medical History: Discussing your medical history and any underlying conditions or medications you're taking can be informative in the diagnostic process.

Comprehensive Metabolic Panel: This blood test assesses various markers, including glucose, insulin, and other metabolic indicators, to gain a comprehensive view of your metabolic health.

Lipid Profile: A lipid profile measures cholesterol levels, including LDL and HDL cholesterol, which can be altered by insulin resistance.

Liver Function Tests: Since insulin resistance can lead to fatty liver disease, assessing liver function can provide insights into associated issues.

It's important to note that a single test may not provide a complete diagnosis of insulin resistance. A healthcare provider may use a combination of these diagnostic tests and assessments to accurately evaluate your insulin sensitivity. Based on the results, they can provide guidance on managing insulin resistance and mitigating its associated health risks.

Understanding the outcomes of diagnostic tests associated with insulin resistance is essential for comprehending your metabolic well-being. Here's a summary of significant figures and their significance:

Fasting Blood Sugar

Normal: Typically, a fasting blood sugar level below 100 milligrams per deciliter (mg/dL) is considered normal.

Pre-Diabetes: Fasting blood sugar levels between 100-125 mg/dL may indicate pre-diabetes.

Diabetes: A fasting blood sugar level of 126 mg/dL or higher on two separate tests is typically indicative of diabetes.

Hemoglobin A1c (HbA1c):

Normal: An HbA1c level of less than 5.7% is considered normal.

Pre-Diabetes: HbA1c levels between 5.7% and 6.4% suggest pre-diabetes.

Diabetes: An HbA1c level of 6.5% or higher is usually indicative of diabetes.

Oral Glucose Tolerance Test (OGTT):

Normal: A two-hour blood sugar level of less than 140 mg/dL is typically considered normal.

Pre-Diabetes: A two-hour blood sugar level between 140-199 mg/dL after an OGTT indicates pre-diabetes.

Diabetes: A two-hour blood sugar level of 200 mg/dL or higher on an OGTT is usually indicative of diabetes.

Insulin Levels

Normal: Fasting insulin levels may vary, but they are typically in the range of 2-25 micro international units per milliliter (µIU/mL).

Insulin Resistance: Elevated fasting insulin levels, especially when accompanied by high blood sugar, can indicate insulin resistance.

Body Measurements

Waist Circumference: In general, a waist circumference of more than 35 inches (88 cm) in women and more than 40 inches (102 cm) in men is associated with an increased risk of insulin resistance.

HDL and LDL Cholesterol:

HDL Cholesterol: Higher levels of HDL (good) cholesterol are desirable, as it can help protect against heart disease.

LDL Cholesterol: Lower levels of LDL (bad) cholesterol are preferred, as high levels are associated with an increased risk of heart disease.

Liver Function Tests

These tests measure various markers, such as alanine transaminase (ALT) and aspartate transaminase (AST), which can indicate liver health. Elevated levels may suggest fatty liver disease associated with insulin resistance.

Hormone Levels (if applicable):

In women with PCOS, hormonal markers such as testosterone and luteinizing hormone (LH) may be assessed.

It's crucial to understand these figures and their significance in managing insulin resistance. If your outcomes suggest insulin resistance or associated health issues, it's essential to work with a healthcare provider to create a customized plan for making lifestyle changes, dietary modifications, and, if required, medical interventions to improve your metabolic health and decrease the risks linked with insulin resistance. Frequently, monitoring and follow-up evaluations are recommended to track progress and make necessary changes to the plan.

Interpreting Blood Sugar and Insulin Levels

Understanding the significance of your blood sugar and insulin levels is key to assessing your metabolic health, particularly in the context of insulin resistance. Here's how to interpret these levels:

Blood Sugar Levels

Fasting Blood Sugar

Normal: Typically, a fasting blood sugar level below 100 milligrams per deciliter (mg/dL) is considered normal. This indicates that your body is effectively regulating blood sugar.

Pre-Diabetes: Fasting blood sugar levels between 100-125 mg/dL may indicate pre-diabetes. It suggests that your body is starting to have trouble regulating blood sugar, and you're at increased risk of developing diabetes.

Diabetes: A fasting blood sugar level of 126 mg/dL or higher on two separate tests is typically indicative of diabetes. This indicates that your body is not effectively regulating blood sugar, and you may require treatment and lifestyle changes.

Hemoglobin A1c (HbA1c)

HbA1c levels

Normal: An HbA1c level of less than 5.7% is considered normal. This indicates that your average blood sugar levels over the past two to three months are within a healthy range.

Pre-Diabetes: HbA1c levels between 5.7% and 6.4% suggest pre-diabetes. This means your average blood sugar levels have been elevated, indicating a risk of progressing to diabetes.

Diabetes: An HbA1c level of 6.5% or higher is usually indicative of diabetes. This suggests that your average blood sugar levels have been consistently high, and you may require treatment and lifestyle changes.

Insulin Levels

Fasting Insulin Levels

Normal: Fasting insulin levels can vary depending on the laboratory, but they are typically in the range of 2-25 micro international units per milliliter (μIU/mL). Normal fasting insulin levels indicate that your body is effectively regulating blood sugar.

Insulin Resistance: Elevated fasting insulin levels, especially when accompanied by high blood sugar, can indicate insulin resistance. This means that your body is producing more insulin to compensate for cells' reduced sensitivity to it.

Interpreting these levels is just the first step. If your results suggest insulin resistance or related health concerns, it's important to work with a healthcare provider. They can help you develop a personalized plan for lifestyle changes, dietary modifications, and, if necessary, medical interventions to improve your metabolic health and reduce the risks associated with insulin resistance. Regular monitoring and follow-up assessments are often recommended to track your progress and make necessary adjustments to your plan.

HbA1c, also known as hemoglobin A1c, is a blood test that provides valuable information about your average blood sugar levels over the past two to three months. It is a critical marker for assessing long-term blood sugar control and is particularly useful in diagnosing and monitoring conditions like diabetes and pre-diabetes. Here's how HbA1c works and why it's important:

Formation of HbA1c

Hemoglobin is a protein found in red blood cells that carries oxygen from the lungs to the body's tissues. When hemoglobin is exposed to glucose (sugar) in the bloodstream, a chemical reaction occurs, resulting in the formation of HbA1c.

Relationship to Blood Sugar

The higher the levels of glucose in your bloodstream, the more glucose binds to hemoglobin. Therefore, HbA1c levels are directly related to your average blood sugar levels over time.

Measure of Long-Term Blood Sugar Control

Unlike a fasting blood sugar test, which provides a snapshot of your blood sugar at a specific moment, HbA1c offers a broader perspective. It reflects your average blood sugar levels over the preceding two to three months. This is important because it accounts for fluctuations in blood sugar that can occur throughout the day and night.

Diagnostic Tool

HbA1c is commonly used to diagnose and classify diabetes and pre-diabetes.

The American Diabetes Association provides the following guidelines:

Normal: HbA1c below 5.7%

Pre-Diabetes: HbA1c between 5.7% and 6.4%

Diabetes: HbA1c of 6.5% or higher on two separate tests

Monitoring Diabetes Control

For individuals with diabetes, HbA1c is a crucial tool for monitoring how well blood sugar levels are being managed. The goal is to keep HbA1c levels within a target range that reduces the risk of complications. The specific target range may vary based on individual factors and the type of diabetes.

Risk Assessment

HbA1c can also help assess the risk of developing diabetes and cardiovascular complications. Elevated HbA1c levels are associated with an increased risk of heart disease.

HbA1c testing is a valuable tool for both diagnosing and managing diabetes. It provides a more comprehensive understanding of long-term blood sugar control compared to other tests that measure blood sugar at a single point in time. Regular monitoring of HbA1c levels is essential for individuals with diabetes to make informed treatment and lifestyle decisions.

Developing a well-rounded eating plan is crucial for managing insulin resistance and promoting overall health. Here is a comprehensive guide to assist you in creating a sustainable and balanced diet:

Seek Professional Assistance

Before making significant dietary changes, it's crucial to consult with a registered dietitian, nutritionist, or healthcare provider who specializes in metabolic health and insulin resistance. They can offer personalized guidance based on your unique requirements and medical history.

Emphasize Whole Foods

Emphasize whole, unprocessed foods in your diet. These include fruits, vegetables, whole grains, lean proteins, and healthy fats. Whole foods are abundant in nutrients and fiber, which can help stabilize blood sugar levels.

Monitor Carbohydrate Intake

Pay attention to the type and amount of carbohydrates you consume. Choose complex carbohydrates, such as whole grains, legumes, and vegetables, which are digested more slowly and have a less dramatic impact on blood sugar. Limit simple sugars and refined carbohydrates, like sugary snacks and white bread.

Control Your Portions

Be mindful of portion sizes to avoid overeating. Use measuring cups or your hand as a reference (e.g., a serving of protein is about the size of your palm).

Aim for Balanced Meals

Strive for balanced meals that include a source of lean protein, healthy fats, and complex carbohydrates. This combination helps maintain steady blood sugar levels.

Choose Healthy Fats

Incorporate healthy fat sources such as avocados, nuts, seeds, and olive oil. These fats can help improve insulin sensitivity.

Include Fiber

High-fiber foods like whole grains, legumes, vegetables, and fruits can slow the absorption of sugar and contribute to better blood sugar control.

Limit Sugary and Processed Foods

Reduce or eliminate sugary snacks, sugary beverages, and heavily processed foods. These can lead to rapid spikes in blood sugar.

Have Balanced Meals Frequently

Eat regular meals and snacks to maintain consistent energy levels and prevent extreme blood sugar fluctuations.

Monitor Blood Sugar Response

Some individuals may benefit from monitoring their blood sugar levels after meals to identify which foods and combinations work best for them. This can help tailor your diet to your specific needs.

Stay Hydrated

Drink plenty of water throughout the day. Dehydration can affect blood sugar control.

Limit Alcohol

If you drink alcohol, do so in moderation, and be aware of its impact on blood sugar.

Time Your Meals

Consider the timing of your meals and snacks. Spacing them evenly throughout the day can help prevent extreme blood sugar fluctuations.

Incorporate Physical Activity

Regular physical activity can improve insulin sensitivity. Incorporate both aerobic exercises and strength training into your routine.

Consistency is Key

Consistency in your eating plan and lifestyle is crucial. Avoid extreme diets or drastic changes. Aim for a sustainable and enjoyable approach to eating.

Tailor Your Plan

Your dietary needs and preferences are unique. Customize your eating plan to suit your taste, cultural background, and dietary restrictions while adhering to the principles of healthy eating.

Regular Follow-Up

Regularly assess your progress and adjust your eating plan as needed. It's essential to work closely with a healthcare provider or registered dietitian for ongoing support.

Remember that managing insulin resistance through diet is a lifelong commitment. A balanced and sustainable eating plan, coupled with a healthy lifestyle, can significantly enhance your metabolic health and decrease the risks associated with insulin resistance.

An insulin-resistant diet is specifically designed to help manage insulin resistance, stabilize blood sugar levels, and promote overall health. It focuses on choosing the right foods and meal timing to improve insulin sensitivity and reduce the risk of associated health problems. Here are the key principles of the insulin-resistance diet:

Balanced Meals

Emphasize balanced meals that include a source of lean protein, healthy fats, and complex carbohydrates. This combination helps maintain steady blood sugar levels.

Choose Whole Foods

Prioritize whole, unprocessed foods. This includes fruits, vegetables, whole grains, legumes, lean proteins, and healthy fats. These foods are rich in nutrients and fiber.

Monitor Carbohydrate Intake

Pay attention to the type and quantity of carbohydrates you consume. Complex carbohydrates, such as whole grains, legumes, and non-starchy vegetables, are preferred. Limit simple sugars and refined carbohydrates.

Fiber-Rich Foods

Include high-fiber foods in your diet. Fiber can slow the absorption of sugar and improve blood sugar control. Whole grains, vegetables, and fruits are excellent sources of fiber.

Portion Control

Be mindful of portion sizes to avoid overeating. This helps with calorie management and blood sugar control.

Healthy Fats

Incorporate sources of healthy fats, like avocados, nuts, seeds, and olive oil. These fats can improve insulin sensitivity.

Limit Sugary and Processed Foods

Minimize or eliminate sugary snacks, sugary beverages, and heavily processed foods. These can lead to rapid blood sugar spikes.

Meal Timing

Consider the timing of your meals and snacks. Spacing them evenly throughout the day can help prevent extreme blood sugar fluctuations.

Regular Meals

Eat regular meals and snacks to maintain consistent energy levels and

prevent extreme blood sugar
fluctuations.

Choose Low-Glycemic Index Foods

- Foods with a low glycemic index (GI) are less likely to cause rapid blood sugar spikes. These include most non-starchy vegetables, legumes, and whole grains.

Monitor Blood Sugar Response

- Some individuals may benefit from monitoring their blood sugar levels after meals to identify which foods and combinations work best for them. This can help tailor your diet to your specific needs.

Hydration

- Stay well-hydrated by drinking plenty of water throughout the day.

Limit Alcohol

- If you consume alcohol, do so in moderation, and be aware of its impact on blood sugar.

Regular Physical Activity

- Incorporate both aerobic exercises and strength training into your routine. Physical activity can improve insulin sensitivity.

Consistency

- Consistency in your eating plan and lifestyle is essential. Avoid extreme diets or drastic changes. Aim for a sustainable and enjoyable approach to eating.

Customization

- Customize your eating plan to suit your taste, cultural background, and dietary restrictions while aligning with the principles of the insulin resistance diet.

It's important to remember that managing insulin resistance through diet is a long-term commitment. A balanced and sustainable eating plan, along with a healthy lifestyle, can significantly improve your metabolic health and reduce the risks associated with insulin resistance. Consulting with a registered dietitian or healthcare provider can provide personalized guidance based on your specific needs.

Key Principles

The key principles for managing insulin resistance and promoting overall metabolic health include:

Balanced Meals Prioritize balanced meals that include a source of lean protein, healthy fats, and complex carbohydrates. This combination helps maintain steady blood sugar levels.

Whole Foods Emphasize whole, unprocessed foods such as fruits, vegetables, whole grains, legumes, lean proteins, and healthy fats. These foods are rich in nutrients and fiber.

Carbohydrate Monitoring Pay attention to the type and quantity of carbohydrates you consume. Complex carbohydrates, like whole grains, legumes, and non-starchy vegetables, are preferred. Limit simple sugars and refined carbohydrates.

Fiber-Rich Diet Include high-fiber foods in your diet. Fiber can slow the absorption of sugar and improve blood sugar control. Whole grains, vegetables, and fruits are excellent sources of fiber.

Portion Control Be mindful of portion sizes to avoid overeating. This helps with calorie management and blood sugar control.

Healthy Fats Incorporate sources of healthy fats, such as avocados, nuts, seeds, and olive oil. These fats can improve insulin sensitivity.

Limit Sugary and Processed Foods Minimize or eliminate sugary snacks, sugary beverages, and heavily processed foods. These can lead to rapid blood sugar spikes.

Meal Timing Consider the timing of your meals and snacks. Spacing them evenly throughout the day can help prevent extreme blood sugar fluctuations.

Regular Meals Eat regular meals and snacks to maintain consistent energy levels and prevent extreme blood sugar fluctuations.

Choose Low-Glycemic Index Foods Foods with a low glycemic index (GI) are less likely to cause rapid blood sugar spikes. These include most non-starchy vegetables, legumes, and whole grains.

Monitoring Blood Sugar Some individuals may benefit from monitoring their blood sugar levels after meals to identify which foods and combinations work best for them. This can help tailor the diet to specific needs.

Hydration Stay well-hydrated by drinking plenty of water throughout the day.

Limit Alcohol If you consume alcohol, do so in moderation, and be aware of its impact on blood sugar.

Regular Physical Activity
Incorporate both aerobic exercises and strength training into your routine. Physical activity can improve insulin sensitivity.

Consistency Maintain consistency in your eating plan and lifestyle. Avoid extreme diets or drastic changes. Aim for a sustainable and enjoyable approach to eating.

Customization Customize your eating plan to suit your taste, cultural background, and dietary restrictions while aligning with the principles of managing insulin resistance.

These principles form the foundation of a healthy lifestyle and eating plan that can help improve insulin sensitivity and reduce the risks associated with insulin resistance. Consulting with a registered dietitian or healthcare provider can provide personalized guidance based on your specific needs and health status.

Foods to Include

When managing insulin resistance, it's important to include foods that can help stabilize blood sugar levels and improve insulin sensitivity. Here are some foods to include in your diet:

Non-Starchy Vegetables

- Leafy greens (spinach, kale, arugula)
- Broccoli
- Cauliflower
- Bell peppers
- Zucchini
- Cucumbers
- Tomatoes
- Brussels sprouts
- Asparagus

Whole Grains

- Oats
- Quinoa
- Brown rice
- Barley
- Whole wheat pasta
- Whole grain bread

Legumes

- Lentils
- Chickpeas
- Black beans
- Kidney beans

Lean Proteins

- Skinless poultry (chicken, turkey)
- Lean cuts of beef or pork
- Fish (salmon, mackerel, trout)
- Tofu
- Tempeh
- Eggs

Healthy Fats

- Avocados
- Nuts (almonds, walnuts, pistachios)
- Seeds (chia, flax, hemp)
- Olive oil
- Fatty fish (salmon, sardines)

Berries

- Blueberries
- Strawberries
- Raspberries
- Blackberries

Low-Fat Dairy or Dairy Alternatives

- Greek yogurt
- Skim milk
- Almond milk
- Soy milk

Herbs and Spices

- Cinnamon
- Turmeric
- Ginger
- Garlic
- Cumin
- Coriander

High-Fiber Foods

- Chia seeds
- Flax seeds
- Psyllium husk
- Bran cereals
- Steel-cut oats

Green Tea

- Green tea contains compounds that may help improve insulin sensitivity.Vinegar:

- Some studies suggest that vinegar, particularly apple cider vinegar, may have a positive impact on blood sugar control.

Including a variety of these foods in your diet can help support better blood sugar regulation and improved insulin sensitivity. It's important to focus on whole, unprocessed foods and maintain a balanced and portion-controlled approach to your meals. Additionally, consult with a registered dietitian or healthcare provider for personalized dietary recommendations based on your specific needs and health status.

Foods to Avoid

When you have insulin resistance, it's important to avoid or limit foods that can cause rapid spikes in blood sugar and contribute to insulin resistance. Here are some foods to avoid or consume in moderation:

Sugary Foods and Beverages

- Soda
- Fruit juices (high in added sugars)
- Candy
- Cookies
- Pastries
- Sugary cereals

Refined Carbohydrates

- White bread

- White rice

- Regular pasta

- Most baked goods made with white flour

Processed and Fast Foods

- Fast food items like burgers and fries
- Frozen dinners high in refined carbohydrates and unhealthy fats
- Highly processed snacks (chips, crackers)

Saturated and Trans Fats

- Fried foods
- Fatty cuts of red meat
- Processed meats (sausages, bacon)

- Margarine and partially hydrogenated oils

Excessive Starchy Vegetables

- While non-starchy vegetables are encouraged, limit starchy ones such as potatoes and corn.

High-Sugar Condiments and Sauces

- Ketchup
- Barbecue sauce
- Sweetened salad dressings

Full-Fat Dairy

- Whole milk

- Full-fat yogurt

- Cream

Excessive Alcohol

- Alcohol can lead to fluctuations in blood sugar. Consume it in moderation.

Sugary Breakfast Cereals

- Many breakfast cereals are high in added sugars.

High-Glycemic Index Foods

- Foods with a high glycemic index can lead to rapid spikes in blood sugar. Limit these, including white potatoes, white rice, and certain breakfast cereals.

Energy Drinks

- These can be high in sugar and caffeine, which may affect blood sugar control.

Artificial Sweeteners

- While artificial sweeteners can be low in calories, some studies suggest they may not be ideal for insulin sensitivity. It's best to use them sparingly or avoid them if they trigger cravings for sugary foods.

Hidden Sugars

- Be cautious of hidden sugars in processed foods. Check ingredient labels for terms like high-fructose corn syrup, cane sugar, and other sweeteners.

It's important to note that individual responses to foods can vary, and what works for one person may not work for another. Maintaining a balanced and personalized diet is key. Consult with a registered dietitian or healthcare provider for specific dietary recommendations based on your unique needs and health status.

To plan your meals effectively for insulin resistance, it's important to create meals that are balanced and nutrient-dense, helping to stabilize blood sugar levels and improve insulin sensitivity. Here's a guide that can help:

Focus on Balanced Meals

Ensure that every meal includes a source of lean protein, healthy fats, and complex carbohydrates. This balance can help regulate blood sugar.

Mind Your Portions

Be aware of portion sizes to avoid overeating. Using smaller plates can help control portions.

Include Non-Starchy Veggies

Non-starchy vegetables, such as leafy greens, broccoli, and bell peppers, should make up a significant portion of your plate. They're low in calories and high in fiber.

Choose Whole Grains

Opt for whole grains like brown rice, quinoa, and whole wheat pasta. They're higher in fiber and nutrients compared to refined grains.

Lean Proteins

Include sources of lean protein, such as skinless poultry, fish, tofu, and legumes. Protein helps maintain fullness and can improve insulin sensitivity.

Healthy Fats

Incorporate healthy fats from sources like avocados, nuts, seeds, and olive oil. These fats can improve insulin sensitivity.

Fiber-Rich Foods

Include high-fiber foods like chia seeds, flax seeds, and legumes. Fibre slows the absorption of sugar and supports blood sugar control.

Limit Simple Sugars

Avoid or reduce foods and drinks high in added sugars, such as sugary snacks, candies, and sweetened drinks.

Regular, Balanced Meals

Try to eat balanced meals and snacks frequently to maintain consistent energy levels and prevent extreme blood sugar fluctuations.

Choose Smart Snacks

Choose healthy snacks like Greek yogurt, nuts, or cut vegetables with hummus to keep blood sugar stable between meals.

Monitor Carbohydrate Intake

Pay attention to the type and amount of carbohydrates you consume. Complex carbohydrates are preferred over simple sugars.

Stay Hydrated

Drink plenty of water throughout the day to help with hydration and blood sugar control.

Meal Timing

Space your meals and snacks evenly throughout the day to maintain consistent energy and blood sugar levels.

Limit Processed Foods

Minimize or eliminate processed and fast foods, which often contain refined carbohydrates and unhealthy fats.

Customize Your Plan

Personalize your meal plan based on your individual preferences, dietary restrictions, and cultural background. Make your meals enjoyable and sustainable.

Consistency is Key

Maintain consistency in your eating plan and lifestyle. Avoid extreme diets or drastic changes.

Regular Physical Activity

Incorporate both aerobic exercises and strength training into your routine. Physical activity can improve insulin sensitivity.

Regular Monitoring

Periodically assess your progress and adjust your meal plan as needed. Consult with a registered dietitian or healthcare provider for ongoing support.

Meal planning for insulin resistance requires a long-term commitment to better health. A balanced and sustainable approach to eating, along with a healthy lifestyle, can significantly improve your metabolic health and reduce the risks associated with insulin resistance.

Hey there! Are you looking to improve your insulin resistance and overall health? Well, building balanced meals is the way to go! Let me walk you through some easy steps to create a well-balanced meal that will provide you with all the essential nutrients your body needs.

First things first, let's add some lean protein to your meal. Whether it's skinless poultry, lean cuts of beef or pork, fish, tofu or legumes like beans and lentils, these are great sources of protein that will keep you feeling full and satisfied.

Next up, let's incorporate some complex carbohydrates like whole grains, starchy vegetables, and legumes. These provide fibre and steady energy to keep you going throughout the day.

Don't forget your non-starchy vegetables! Fill up a significant portion of your plate with leafy greens, broccoli, cauliflower, and bell peppers. They are low in calories and rich in vitamins and minerals, making them an excellent addition to any meal.

Healthy fats are also important, so make sure to add sources like avocados, nuts, seeds, and olive oil to your meals. These fats are heart-healthy and can help improve insulin sensitivity.

Fiber is also a crucial part of balanced meals, so choose high-fiber foods like whole grains, legumes, and vegetables. Fiber can help regulate blood sugar levels and promote fullness, so you won't feel hungry soon after eating.

Remember, portion control is key, so be mindful of the amount of food you're consuming. Use measuring cups or your hand as a reference to avoid overeating.

The flavor of your meals matters too! Season your meals with herbs and spices instead of excess salt or sugar to enhance the flavor without adding unhealthy ingredients.

Don't forget to stay hydrated by drinking water with your meals, as dehydration can affect blood sugar control.

Spacing your meals and snacks evenly throughout the day can help maintain consistent energy levels and prevent extreme blood sugar fluctuations. And if you need a snack, healthy options like Greek yoghurt, nuts, or cut vegetables with hummus can help stabilize blood sugar levels.

Minimize or eliminate processed and fast foods, which often contain refined carbohydrates and unhealthy fats. And customize your meals to suit your preferences, dietary restrictions, and cultural background. Personalizing your meals will make them enjoyable and sustainable.

Regular physical activity is also essential, so incorporate both aerobic exercises and strength training into your routine. Physical activity can improve insulin sensitivity and overall health.

Periodically assess your dietary habits and adjust your meal planning as needed. Consult with a registered dietitian or healthcare provider for ongoing support.

By following these guidelines and building balanced meals, you can better manage insulin resistance, support your metabolic health, and reduce the risks associated with insulin resistance. So why not give it a try? Your body will thank you!

Here are some sample meal plans for managing insulin resistance. These are just examples, and it's important to customize your meal plans to fit your individual preferences and dietary needs. Consult with a registered dietitian or healthcare provider for personalized guidance.

Sample Meal Plan

Breakfast

Scrambled eggs with spinach and tomatoes

Whole-grain toast

A small apple

Lunch

Grilled chicken breast salad with mixed greens, cucumbers, and a vinaigrette dressing

Quinoa on the side

Snack

Greek yogurt with berries and a drizzle of honey

Dinner

Baked salmon with lemon and herbs

Steamed broccoli

Brown rice

Sample Meal Plan

Breakfast

Oatmeal with sliced almonds and blueberries

A boiled egg

Green tea

Lunch

Lentil and vegetable soup

Mixed green salad with balsamic vinaigrette

Snack

Carrot and cucumber sticks with hummus

Dinner

Stir-fried tofu with mixed vegetables
(broccoli, bell peppers, snap peas) in a
light teriyaki sauce

Quinoa

Sample Meal Plan

Breakfast

Greek yogurt parfait with granola and
fresh strawberries

Lunch

Turkey and avocado wrap with whole
wheat tortilla

Side of mixed greens

Snack

A handful of mixed nuts

Dinner

Grilled shrimp with garlic and herbs

Roasted asparagus

Mashed cauliflower

Sample Meal Plan (Vegetarian)

Breakfast

Smoothie with spinach, banana, almond milk, and chia seeds

Lunch

Chickpea and vegetable curry

Brown rice

Snack

Sliced bell peppers with guacamole

Dinner

Baked sweet potato with black beans, salsa, and a dollop of Greek yogurt

Remember to monitor your portion sizes, stay well-hydrated with water, and adjust these meal plans to suit your calorie and nutritional needs. The goal is to create balanced meals that provide a combination of protein, healthy fats, complex carbohydrates, and plenty of non-starchy vegetables to help manage insulin resistance and maintain overall health.

Nutritional strategies for managing insulin resistance focus on making informed choices about the foods you eat and how you structure your meals. Here are some key nutritional strategies to help improve insulin sensitivity and regulate blood sugar levels:

Choose Complex Carbohydrates

Prioritize complex carbohydrates like whole grains (e.g., brown rice, quinoa, whole wheat), legumes, and non-starchy vegetables. These carbohydrates are digested more slowly, preventing rapid blood sugar spikes.

Monitor Carbohydrate Intake

Pay attention to the quantity and type of carbohydrates in your meals. Avoid excessive consumption of simple sugars, refined carbohydrates, and high-glycemic index foods.

Prioritize Lean Proteins

Include lean sources of protein in your diet, such as skinless poultry, fish, lean cuts of meat, tofu, and legumes. Protein helps maintain fullness and supports blood sugar control.

Healthy Fats

Incorporate sources of healthy fats like avocados, nuts, seeds, and olive oil. These fats can improve insulin sensitivity and provide essential nutrients.

High-Fiber Foods

Choose foods high in fiber, such as whole grains, legumes, and non-starchy vegetables. Fiber slows the absorption of sugar and supports better blood sugar regulation.

Balanced Meals

Create balanced meals that include a combination of protein, carbohydrates, and fats. This helps maintain stable blood sugar levels.

Portion Control

Be mindful of portion sizes to avoid overeating. Measuring and controlling portions can help with calorie management and blood sugar control.

Meal Timing

Space your meals and snacks evenly throughout the day to prevent extreme blood sugar fluctuations.

Snack Smart

If needed, include healthy snacks between meals, like Greek yogurt, nuts, or cut vegetables with hummus, to maintain stable blood sugar levels.

Avoid Sugary and Processed Foods

- Minimize or eliminate sugary snacks, sugary beverages, and heavily processed foods, which can lead to rapid blood sugar spikes.

Limit Simple Sugars

- Reduce your intake of foods and beverages high in added sugars, as they can disrupt blood sugar control.

Hydration

- Stay well-hydrated by drinking water throughout the day. Dehydration can affect blood sugar control.

Customize Your Plan

- Tailor your nutritional strategies to your personal preferences, dietary restrictions, and cultural background. Make your eating plan enjoyable and sustainable.

Regular Physical Activity

- Incorporate both aerobic exercises and strength training into your routine. Regular physical activity can improve insulin sensitivity.

Consistency

- Maintain consistency in your dietary habits and lifestyle. Avoid extreme diets or drastic changes.

Regular Monitoring

- Periodically assess your dietary habits and adjust your nutritional strategies as needed. Consult with a registered dietitian or healthcare provider for ongoing support.

These nutritional strategies are essential for managing insulin resistance and promoting overall metabolic health. A balanced and sustainable approach to eating, along with a healthy lifestyle, can significantly reduce the risks associated with insulin resistance.

Carbohydrates play a crucial role in managing insulin resistance, as they have a direct impact on blood sugar levels and insulin sensitivity. Understanding the types of carbohydrates and how they affect your body is essential when dealing with insulin resistance:

Complex Carbohydrates

Complex carbohydrates, found in foods like whole grains, legumes, and non-starchy vegetables, are composed of longer chains of sugar molecules. They are digested more slowly, leading to a gradual and moderate increase in blood sugar. This slow digestion helps prevent blood sugar spikes and is beneficial for individuals with insulin resistance.

Simple Carbohydrates

Simple carbohydrates, on the other hand, are composed of one or two sugar molecules and are found in foods like table sugar, honey, and sugary snacks. They are quickly digested and cause rapid spikes in blood sugar levels. It's best to limit or avoid simple carbohydrates to manage insulin resistance.

Glycemic Index (GI)

The glycemic index measures how quickly a carbohydrate-containing food raises blood sugar levels. Foods with a high GI cause rapid spikes in blood sugar, while those with a low GI lead to a slower and more gradual increase. Managing insulin resistance often involves choosing foods with a low to moderate GI to prevent blood sugar fluctuations.

Portion Control

Controlling the quantity of carbohydrates you consume is essential. Even complex carbohydrates can impact blood sugar if consumed in large quantities. Pay attention to portion sizes to manage calorie intake and blood sugar levels.

Balancing Macronutrients

Creating balanced meals that include a combination of carbohydrates, protein, and healthy fats can help maintain stable blood sugar levels. The presence of protein and fats can slow down the absorption of carbohydrates, preventing rapid blood sugar spikes.

Individual Variation

It's important to note that individual responses to carbohydrates can vary. What works for one person may not work for another. Monitoring your blood sugar response to different foods can help you tailor your carbohydrate intake to your specific needs.

Fiber Content

Foods high in fiber, such as whole grains, legumes, and non-starchy vegetables, can help regulate blood sugar levels. Fiber slows the digestion of carbohydrates and provides a feeling of fullness.

Customization

Customize your carbohydrate intake to fit your personal preferences and dietary restrictions. Make choices that you find enjoyable and sustainable.

Managing carbohydrates is a key component of a dietary plan for insulin resistance. By focusing on complex carbohydrates, controlling portion sizes, and paying attention to the glycemic index, you can regulate blood sugar levels, improve insulin sensitivity, and reduce the risks associated with insulin resistance. Consulting with a registered dietitian or healthcare provider can provide personalized guidance based on your specific needs and health status.

Complex vs. Simple Carbs

Understanding the difference between complex and simple carbohydrates is crucial for managing insulin resistance. Here's a breakdown of these two types of carbs and their impact on insulin and blood sugar:

Complex Carbohydrates

Structure: Complex carbohydrates are composed of long chains of sugar molecules, which take longer to break down in the digestive system.

Food Sources: They are found in foods such as whole grains (e.g., brown rice, whole wheat bread, oats), legumes (beans, lentils), and non-starchy vegetables (e.g., broccoli, spinach).

Impact on Blood Sugar: Complex carbs are digested slowly, leading to a gradual increase in blood sugar levels. They help maintain stable blood sugar levels and are often recommended for individuals with insulin resistance.

Fibre Content: Many complex carbohydrate sources are rich in fiber, which further slows digestion and promotes fullness.

Simple Carbohydrates

Structure: Simple carbohydrates are composed of one or two sugar molecules, making them easy to digest.

Food Sources: They are found in foods like table sugar, honey, fruit juices, candies, and sugary snacks.

Impact on Blood Sugar: Simple carbs are rapidly digested and cause a quick spike in blood sugar levels. They are not ideal for individuals with insulin resistance, as they can lead to blood sugar fluctuations.

Glycemic Index: Simple carbohydrates are often associated with a high glycemic index (GI), indicating their ability to cause rapid blood sugar spikes.

For managing insulin resistance, it's important to prioritize complex carbohydrates over simple ones. Complex carbs are generally digested more slowly, which helps prevent blood sugar spikes and provides a steadier source of energy. Additionally, foods high in fibre, like whole grains and non-starchy vegetables, can enhance insulin sensitivity and support better blood sugar control.

While avoiding simple carbohydrates is advisable, it's also essential to monitor portion sizes, as even complex carbohydrates can affect blood sugar levels if consumed in excess. Balancing carbohydrates with protein and healthy fats in your meals can further aid in stabilizing blood sugar and improving insulin sensitivity.

Customizing your carbohydrate intake to fit your specific dietary preferences and needs, and consulting with a registered dietitian or healthcare provider for personalized guidance, can help you effectively manage insulin resistance through your carbohydrate choices.

The Glycemic Index

The Glycemic Index (GI) ranks carbohydrate-containing foods based on how quickly and to what extent they raise blood sugar levels after being consumed. It assigns a numerical value to different foods, indicating their impact on blood sugar. Here are some key things to know about the Glycemic Index

Scale

The GI scale ranges from 0 to 100, with pure glucose having a GI of 100. Glucose serves as the point of reference since it raises blood sugar the fastest.

Categories

Low, medium, and high GI categories are used to classify foods according to their impact on blood sugar:

Low GI (0-55): These foods have a slower and steadier effect on blood sugar and are beneficial for insulin-resistant individuals.

Medium GI (56-69): Foods in this category have a moderate impact on blood sugar and can be consumed in moderation.

High GI (70 or above): High-GI foods cause a rapid spike in blood sugar and should be limited, particularly for those with insulin resistance.

Factors Influencing GI

Various factors influence the GI of a food, including the type of carbohydrate, processing, cooking methods, and the presence of fiber and fat. Foods that contain fiber, protein, and fat tend to have a lower GI.

Role in Insulin Resistance

Understanding the GI of foods can aid insulin-resistant individuals. Opting for low-GI foods can help stabilize blood sugar levels and reduce the risk of blood sugar spikes.

Using the GI

Although the GI is a useful tool, it's critical to consider the overall meal composition. Combining low-GI foods with protein, healthy fats, and non-starchy vegetables can further improve blood sugar control.

Limitations

The GI does not account for portion sizes, which can significantly affect blood sugar response. Therefore, it's important to consider both the GI and portion control for effective blood sugar management.

Customization

The GI of foods can differ among individuals. Foods that have a high GI for one person may not have the same impact on another. As a result, it's important to take into account your response to different foods.

Whole Foods

Whole, unprocessed foods, such as whole grains, non-starchy vegetables, and legumes, typically have a lower GI compared to highly processed and refined foods.

Using the GI as a tool, alongside portion control and balanced meal planning, can assist insulin-resistant individuals in making informed decisions about the carbohydrates they consume. Prioritizing foods with a lower GI can lead to better blood sugar control and improved insulin sensitivity.

Proteins and Fats

Proteins and fats are essential macronutrients that play a significant role in managing insulin resistance. Understanding how to include the right types and amounts of proteins and fats in your diet can help improve insulin sensitivity and overall metabolic health. Here's what you need to know about proteins and fats

Proteins

Role in Insulin Resistance

Protein is essential for maintaining and repairing tissues, and it plays a role in insulin sensitivity. Including adequate protein in your diet can help regulate blood sugar levels and improve satiety.

Sources of Lean Protein

Choose lean sources of protein to reduce saturated fat intake. Options include skinless poultry, fish, lean cuts of beef or pork, tofu,

tempeh, legumes (beans, lentils), and low-fat
dairy products.

Portion Control

Be mindful of portion sizes. A typical serving of
lean protein is about the size of your palm.
Balancing protein with carbohydrates and fats
in your meals can help stabilize blood sugar
levels.

Protein and Satiety

Protein-rich foods tend to keep you feeling full
for longer, which can help prevent overeating
and stabilize your energy levels.

Fats

Role in Insulin Resistance

Healthy fats are important for overall health,
and they can improve insulin sensitivity. They
are essential for the absorption of fat-soluble

vitamins and the maintenance of cell membranes.

Sources of Healthy Fats

Include sources of healthy fats in your diet, such as avocados, nuts (e.g., almonds, walnuts, pistachios), seeds (e.g., chia seeds, flaxseeds, hemp seeds), olive oil, and fatty fish (e.g., salmon, mackerel, trout).

Limit Saturated and Trans Fats

Avoid or minimize saturated fats found in fried foods, fatty cuts of red meat, and processed meats (like sausages and bacon). Additionally, avoid trans fats, often found in partially hydrogenated oils and many processed foods.

Balancing Fats

A well-balanced diet includes a mix of different types of fats, including monounsaturated fats (e.g., in olive oil), polyunsaturated fats (e.g., in fatty fish and some seeds), and a limited amount of saturated fats.

Portion Control

While healthy fats are beneficial, they are calorie-dense. Be mindful of portion sizes, and aim for moderation.

Omega-3 Fatty Acids

Omega-3 fatty acids, found in fatty fish and certain seeds, may have additional benefits for insulin sensitivity and heart health.

Cooking Methods

Use healthy cooking methods like grilling, baking, and sautéing rather than deep-frying to limit added fats.

Balancing proteins and fats in your diet is essential for managing insulin resistance. Lean protein sources and healthy fats can help stabilize blood sugar levels and improve overall metabolic health. It's important to create meals that include a balance of all macronutrients, along with non-starchy vegetables and complex carbohydrates, for optimal blood sugar control.

Customizing your protein and fat intake based on your dietary preferences and needs can make it easier to maintain a healthy and enjoyable eating plan.

Choosing Healthy Sources

Choosing healthy sources of proteins and fats is crucial for managing insulin resistance and promoting overall health. Here are some tips on how to select nutritious sources of these macronutrients:

Healthy Sources of Proteins

Lean Meats: Opt for lean cuts of meat, such as skinless poultry (chicken, turkey), lean cuts of beef or pork, and trimmed cuts of lamb. These choices provide protein without excess saturated fat.

Fatty Fish: Include fatty fish like salmon, mackerel, trout, and sardines. They are rich in omega-3 fatty acids, which can improve insulin sensitivity.

Plant-Based Proteins: Incorporate plant-based protein sources, such as tofu, tempeh, legumes (beans, lentils, chickpeas), and edamame. These options are low in saturated fat and provide fiber.

Low-Fat Dairy: If you consume dairy, choose low-fat or fat-free options like Greek yoghurt and skim milk. They are sources of protein without the added saturated fat found in whole dairy products.

Poultry without Skin: When enjoying chicken or turkey, remove the skin to reduce saturated fat content while retaining protein.

Eggs: Eggs are a good source of protein. You can include them in your diet, but consider preparing them with minimal added fat (e.g., scrambled without excessive butter or oil).

Healthy Sources of Fats

Avocados are rich in monounsaturated fats and provide essential nutrients. They can be added to salads, sandwiches, or used as a healthy spread.

Nuts and Seeds Incorporate nuts (almonds, walnuts, pistachios) and seeds (chia seeds, flaxseeds, hemp seeds) as snacks or toppings for oatmeal and yogurt. They are sources of healthy fats and fiber.

Olive Oil Use extra-virgin olive oil for salad dressings and light sautéing. It's a monounsaturated fat that's heart-healthy.

Fatty Fish Fatty fish like salmon, mackerel, and sardines are excellent sources of omega-3 fatty acids, which have anti-inflammatory properties and may enhance insulin sensitivity.

Nut Butter Opt for natural nut kinds of butter without added sugars or hydrogenated oils. Peanut, almond, and cashew jars of butter can be spread on whole-grain toast or used in smoothies.

Coconut Oil While coconut oil has gained popularity, it's higher in saturated fat. Use it sparingly or consider alternatives like olive oil or canola oil.

Low-Fat Dairy If you consume dairy, choose low-fat or fat-free options for reduced saturated fat content.

Dark Chocolate Dark chocolate with a high cocoa content can be a treat in moderation. It contains antioxidants and healthy fats.

Remember that the key to managing insulin resistance is balance and moderation. Customizing your diet to include a variety of these healthy protein and fat sources, along with complex carbohydrates, non-starchy vegetables, and fiber, can support better blood sugar control and overall metabolic health. Consulting with a registered dietitian can provide personalized guidance based on your specific dietary preferences and needs.

Portion Control

Portion control is an essential aspect of managing insulin resistance and supporting better blood sugar control. Regulating the size of your portions can help you manage your calorie intake, prevent overeating, and avoid sudden spikes in blood sugar. Here are some tips for effective portion control.

Use Measuring Tools

Measuring cups, kitchen scales, and measuring spoons can assist you in accurately portioning your food, especially when you're learning proper portion sizes.

Learn Visual Cues

Visual cues can help you develop a sense of portion sizes over time. For instance, a deck of cards can represent an appropriate portion size for meat, poultry, or fish.

Half Your Plate

When creating meals, aim to fill half of your plate with non-starchy vegetables. This helps you control the portion sizes of more calorie-dense foods.

Mindful Eating

Pay attention to hunger and fullness cues. Eat slowly, savor your food, and stop when you're satisfied, rather than when you're overly full.

Smaller Plates and Bowls

Using smaller dishes can create the illusion of a fuller plate, which can be helpful for portion control.

Read Food Labels

Check food labels for serving sizes to be aware of how much you're consuming. Sometimes, a package may contain multiple servings.

Avoid "Supersizing

When dining out, resist the temptation to upgrade to larger portion sizes. Stick with standard servings.

Share or Pack Leftovers

If the portion is too large when dining out, consider sharing with a friend or taking part of it home for another meal.

Plan Snacks

Pre-portioning snacks into small containers or bags can prevent overeating.

Be Mindful of Liquid Calories

Be cautious of beverages like sugary sodas and fruit juices, as liquid calories can add up quickly. Opt for water, unsweetened tea, or other low-calorie drinks.

Track Your Intake

Consider using a food diary or a mobile app to record your meals and portion sizes. This can help you become more aware of your eating habits.

Listen to Hunger and Fullness Signals

Pay attention to your body's signals. Eat when you're hungry and stop when you're satisfied, rather than eating for emotional reasons or boredom.

Avoid Eating Straight from Containers

Instead of eating directly from a bag or box, portion your food onto a plate. This can help you be more aware of how much you're consuming.

Effective portion control is a valuable tool for managing insulin resistance. It allows you to manage your calorie intake, maintain stable blood sugar levels, and support your overall health. With practice, it can become a natural part of your eating habits. Consulting with a registered dietitian can provide additional guidance and support for implementing effective portion control strategies in your daily life.

Fiber and Insulin Sensitivity

Fibre plays a significant role in improving insulin sensitivity and managing insulin resistance. Here's how fiber benefits your metabolic health:

Stabilizes Blood Sugar

Dietary fiber, particularly soluble fiber, helps regulate blood sugar levels by slowing the absorption of carbohydrates. This prevents rapid spikes in blood sugar after meals, which is crucial for individuals with insulin resistance.

Enhances Satiety

High-fiber foods tend to be more filling, which can help with appetite control and weight management. Maintaining a healthy weight is key to improving insulin sensitivity.

Supports Healthy Gut Bacteria

Fiber acts as a prebiotic, providing nourishment for beneficial gut bacteria. A balanced gut microbiome is linked to improved metabolic health and reduced inflammation.

Reduces Inflammation

Chronic inflammation is associated with insulin resistance and related metabolic issues. Fiber-rich foods can help reduce inflammation in the body.

Promotes Weight Management

Fiber-rich foods often have fewer calories and can help with weight loss or maintenance. Excess body weight is a risk factor for insulin resistance.

Lowers LDL Cholesterol

Soluble fiber can help reduce low-density lipoprotein (LDL) cholesterol levels, contributing to better heart health. Heart health is closely linked to metabolic health.

Improves Digestive Health

Fiber prevents constipation and supports a healthy digestive system. A well-functioning digestive system is important for overall well-being.

Encourages a Balanced Diet

Many high-fiber foods, like whole grains, legumes, fruits, and vegetables, are also rich in essential nutrients. Consuming a variety of fiber sources can contribute to a well-rounded diet.

To increase your fiber intake and improve insulin sensitivity

Include Whole Grains Opt for whole grains like brown rice, quinoa, whole wheat, and oats in place of refined grains.

Eat More Fruits and Vegetables Consume a variety of non-starchy vegetables and fruits, as they are excellent sources of fiber.

Choose Legumes Incorporate beans, lentils, chickpeas, and other legumes into your meals.

Snack on Nuts and Seeds Enjoy small portions of nuts and seeds as snacks or additions to meals.

Gradual Increase If you're not used to a high-fiber diet, gradually increase your fiber intake to allow your digestive system to adjust.

Stay Hydrated Ensure you drink enough water along with a high-fiber diet to prevent constipation.

Fiber is a valuable tool for improving insulin sensitivity and overall metabolic health. By incorporating fiber-rich foods into your daily meals and snacks, you can support better blood sugar control and reduce the risks associated with insulin resistance.

Benefits of Fiber

Fiber has a broad range of health advantages and is vital for various aspects of overall well-being. Here are the primary benefits of adding fiber to your diet:

Enhanced Digestive Health

Dietary fiber helps to promote regular bowel movements, prevent constipation, and maintain a healthy digestive system. It adds bulk to stool and softens it, making it easier to pass.

Management of Weight

Foods high in fiber tend to be more filling and can help control appetite, reducing the likelihood of overeating. This can be beneficial for weight management and preventing obesity.

Regulation of Blood Sugar

Soluble fiber can slow down the digestion and absorption of carbohydrates, leading to better blood sugar control. It is particularly important for individuals with diabetes or insulin resistance.

Lowering Cholesterol Levels

Soluble fiber can assist in lowering LDL (low-density lipoprotein) cholesterol levels, which is associated with a lower risk of heart disease.

Heart Health

A diet rich in fiber is connected to improved heart health, as it can help lower blood pressure, reduce inflammation, and support overall cardiovascular well-being.

Healthy Gut Bacteria

Fiber acts as a prebiotic, nourishing beneficial gut bacteria. A balanced and diverse gut microbiome is associated with various health benefits.

Reduced Risk of Colon Cancer

A high-fiber diet may decrease the risk of colorectal cancer by promoting healthy bowel movements and reducing exposure to potentially harmful substances in the colon.

Enhanced Satiety

Foods high in fiber provide a feeling of fullness, which can help with portion control and overall calorie intake.

Reduced Risk of Diverticular Disease

A fiber-rich diet can lower the risk of diverticulitis and diverticular disease, conditions that affect the colon.

Improved Nutrient Absorption

- Some types of fiber can slow down nutrient absorption, which can be beneficial for individuals who need to manage their blood sugar levels or have specific dietary requirements.

Lowered Risk of Hemorrhoids

- Fiber helps prevent constipation, which can decrease the risk of developing painful hemorrhoids.

Management of Metabolic Conditions

- Consuming fiber is beneficial for individuals with metabolic conditions such as insulin resistance, prediabetes, and type 2 diabetes.

It's important to understand that there are two primary types of dietary fiber: soluble and insoluble. Each kind has slightly different properties and health benefits. A well-balanced diet should include both types of fiber from various food sources, such as whole grains, fruits, vegetables, legumes, nuts, and seeds. Adjusting your fiber intake to fit your dietary preferences and needs can help you enjoy these health benefits while promoting overall well-being.

High-Fiber Foods

It is crucial to include high-fiber foods in your diet if you want to improve your health, manage your weight, and maintain better blood sugar control, particularly if you have insulin resistance. The following is a list of high-fiber foods to consider incorporating into your meals:

Whole grains

Brown rice

Quinoa

Steel-cut or old-fashioned oats

Whole wheat pasta

Barley

Whole grain bread (check for high-fiber content)

Legumes

Lentils

Garbanzo beans (chickpeas)

Black beans

Kidney beans

Pinto beans

Vegetables

Broccoli

Spinach

Brussels sprouts

Cauliflower

Carrots

Bell peppers

Sweet potatoes

Zucchini

Kale

Fruits

Apples

Pears

Berries (strawberries, blueberries, raspberries)

Oranges

Bananas

Prunes

Kiwifruit

Avocado

Nuts and seeds

Almonds

Chia seeds

Flaxseeds

Sunflower seeds

Pumpkin seeds

Bran cereals

Bran flakes

Wheat bran

Oatmeal

Choose whole oats or steel-cut oats for higher fiber content.

Popcorn

Air-popped or lightly seasoned popcorn is a good source of dietary fiber.

Whole grain pasta

Whole wheat pasta or pasta made from alternative grains like lentil or chickpea pasta.

High-fiber snacks

Snack on raw vegetables with hummus or choose whole-grain crackers with nut butter.

Edamame

Edamame (young soybeans) is a protein-rich and high-fiber snack.

High-fiber cereals

Look for cereals with at least 5 grams of fiber per serving.

When incorporating high-fiber foods into your diet, remember to gradually increase your fiber intake if you're not used to consuming a lot of fiber. This can help your digestive system adapt. Additionally, make sure to drink plenty of water as fiber absorbs water, which can help maintain proper hydration.

Aim to create balanced meals that include a variety of high-fiber foods, such as whole grains, lean proteins, healthy fats, and non-starchy vegetables. This approach will support better blood sugar control and overall metabolic health. If you want personalized guidance on how to effectively include high-fiber foods in your diet, consider consulting with a registered dietitian.

Lifestyle and Insulin Resistance

Lifestyle plays a significant role in the development and management of insulin resistance. Making positive lifestyle choices can have a substantial impact on your overall metabolic health. Here are key lifestyle factors to consider when addressing insulin resistance:

Diet

Balanced Nutrition: Consume a well-balanced diet rich in whole grains, lean proteins, healthy fats, and high-fiber foods like fruits and vegetables. Avoid or limit processed foods, sugary beverages, and excessive simple carbohydrates.

Portion Control: Practice portion control to manage calorie intake and blood sugar levels. This is essential for weight management and preventing blood sugar spikes.

Regular Meals: Eat regular, balanced meals and avoid skipping meals, which can lead to overeating and blood sugar imbalances.

Hydration: Stay well-hydrated by drinking water throughout the day. Dehydration can affect blood sugar control.

Physical Activity

Regular Exercise: Incorporate regular physical activity into your routine. Both aerobic exercises (e.g., walking, jogging, swimming) and strength training can improve insulin sensitivity.

Consistency: Maintain a consistent exercise routine. Aim for at least 150 minutes of moderate-intensity aerobic activity per week, as recommended by health guidelines.

Weight Management

Maintain a Healthy Weight: Achieving and maintaining a healthy weight is vital for managing insulin resistance. Even a modest weight loss can significantly improve insulin sensitivity.

Stress Management

Stress Reduction: Chronic stress can impact insulin sensitivity. Incorporate stress reduction techniques such as mindfulness, meditation, yoga, or deep breathing exercises into your daily life.

Sleep

Adequate Sleep: Aim for 7-9 hours of quality sleep per night. Poor sleep can affect hormone regulation and insulin sensitivity.

Smoking and Alcohol

Avoid Smoking: Smoking is associated with an increased risk of insulin resistance and type 2 diabetes. Quitting smoking can improve your metabolic health.

Limit Alcohol: If you drink alcohol, do so in moderation. Excessive alcohol consumption can affect blood sugar control.

Regular Check-Ups

Health Monitoring: Schedule regular check-ups with your healthcare provider. Monitoring your blood sugar levels, blood pressure, and cholesterol is essential for early detection and management of metabolic issues.

Medication Management

Medication Compliance: If you have diabetes or other medical conditions that require medication, adhere to your prescribed treatment plan and consult your healthcare provider regularly.

Support and Education

Disease Management: Educate yourself about insulin resistance and its management. Seek support from healthcare professionals, registered dietitians, or support groups to help you make informed decisions.

Individualized Approach

Customization: Your lifestyle choices should be tailored to your specific needs and preferences. What works for one person may not work for another. Consult with healthcare professionals for personalized guidance.

Addressing insulin resistance through lifestyle changes is a holistic approach that can lead to significant improvements in your metabolic health. By combining a balanced diet, regular exercise, stress management, and other positive lifestyle choices, you can effectively manage insulin resistance and reduce the risks associated with this condition.

Exercise and Physical Activity

Exercise and physical activity are essential components of managing insulin resistance and improving overall metabolic health. Regular physical activity can help enhance insulin sensitivity, lower blood sugar levels, and support weight management. Here are key points to consider regarding exercise and physical activity:

Aerobic Exercise

Aerobic activities like brisk walking, jogging, cycling, and swimming can help lower blood sugar levels. Aim for at least 150 minutes of moderate-intensity aerobic exercise per week, as recommended by health guidelines.

Strength Training

Incorporate strength training exercises at least two days a week. Building muscle can improve insulin sensitivity and boost metabolism.

Consistency

Consistency in your exercise routine is key. Regular, ongoing physical activity provides the most significant benefits for managing insulin resistance.

Individualized Approach

Your exercise program should be tailored to your fitness level and preferences. Consult with a healthcare provider or a fitness professional to create a personalized plan.

Post-Meal Activity

Short walks after meals can help regulate blood sugar levels. Consider a 10-15 minute walk following lunch or dinner.

Enjoyable Activities

Choose physical activities you enjoy to make
exercise a sustainable part of your lifestyle.
This can include dancing, gardening, or
recreational sports.

Stress Reduction

Physical activity can also help reduce stress,
which is important for insulin sensitivity.
Activities like yoga or tai chi can combine
exercise and stress management.

Safety Precautions

If you have underlying health conditions,
consult with a healthcare provider before
starting a new exercise program to ensure it's
safe for you.

Tracking Progress

Keep track of your exercise routine and progress. Monitoring your achievements can be motivating.

Support and Accountability

Consider exercising with a friend or joining a fitness class for added motivation and accountability.

Rest and Recovery

Adequate rest and recovery are essential for injury prevention and overall health. Listen to your body and allow time for recovery between intense workouts.

Consultation

Seek guidance from a registered dietitian or healthcare provider who can provide recommendations specific to your needs and health status.

Exercise, when combined with dietary changes
and other positive lifestyle habits, is a powerful
tool for managing insulin resistance. It can
improve insulin sensitivity, promote weight
management, and reduce the risks associated
with metabolic conditions like type 2 diabetes.
Making exercise a regular part of your life is an
investment in your long-term health and
well-being.

The Role of Exercise

Managing insulin resistance is significantly improved with regular exercise as it positively affects the body's insulin response and blood sugar levels. Here is how exercise can influence insulin sensitivity and improve overall metabolic health:

Better Insulin Sensitivity

Physical activity improves the body's ability to efficiently use insulin. When you engage in exercise, your muscle cells become more responsive to insulin, allowing for better uptake and utilization of glucose.

Lowered Blood Sugar Levels

Consistent exercise can help reduce blood sugar levels, especially after meals. This is important for individuals with insulin resistance as it helps prevent blood sugar spikes and maintains stable levels.

Weight Control

Exercise is beneficial for weight loss and helps maintain a healthy weight. Excess body weight is a significant risk factor for insulin resistance, and losing even a small amount of weight can improve insulin sensitivity.

Increased Muscle Mass

Strength training and resistance exercises can increase muscle mass. Muscles are more metabolically active, which can contribute to better blood sugar control.

Improved Lipid Profile

Exercise can lower triglycerides and increase high-density lipoprotein (HDL) cholesterol levels, which promote heart health and metabolic well-being.

Enhanced Cardiovascular Health

Regular exercise can strengthen the heart, lower blood pressure, and reduce the risk of cardiovascular diseases, which often co-occur with insulin resistance.

Stress Reduction

Physical activity can be an effective tool for managing stress. Chronic stress is associated with insulin resistance, so exercise's stress-reduction benefits are valuable.

Better Blood Circulation

Exercise improves blood circulation, allowing for more effective delivery of nutrients and oxygen to cells and removal of waste products.

Post-Meal Advantages

Taking short walks or doing light exercises after meals can help stabilize post-meal blood sugar levels.

Long-Term Health Benefits

- Regular exercise can lower the risk of developing type 2 diabetes and can be a part of a comprehensive strategy for managing existing diabetes.

Customization

- Your exercise routine should be tailored to your preferences and fitness level. The most effective exercise is the one you enjoy and can sustain over the long term.

Consultation

- Before starting a new exercise program, especially if you have underlying health conditions or are new to exercise, consult with a healthcare provider.

Consistency

- Consistency in your exercise routine is essential for achieving long-term benefits.

Incorporating exercise into your lifestyle
regularly is crucial.

By incorporating exercise into your daily
routine along with a balanced diet, you can
manage insulin resistance effectively. It can
significantly improve insulin sensitivity, help
maintain a healthy weight, and reduce the risks
associated with metabolic conditions. Whether
you choose aerobic activities, strength training,
or a combination of both, the positive effects of
exercise on insulin sensitivity are
well-established and provide numerous health
benefits.

Creating an Exercise Routine

Creating an exercise routine that suits your needs and preferences is essential for managing insulin resistance and improving your overall health. Here are steps to help you develop an effective exercise plan:

Set Clear Goals

Define your specific fitness and health goals. Are you aiming for better blood sugar control, weight loss, muscle strength, or overall well-being?

Consult a Healthcare Provider

Before starting any new exercise program, especially if you have underlying health conditions, consult with your healthcare provider to ensure that your plan is safe and appropriate for your individual situation.

Choose Activities You Enjoy

Select exercises and physical activities that you genuinely enjoy. Whether it's walking, cycling, swimming, dancing, or a team sport, finding activities you like makes it more likely that you'll stick with your routine.

Schedule Regular Workouts

Consistency is key. Plan regular workouts and set a schedule that you can realistically follow. Aim for at least 150 minutes of moderate-intensity aerobic exercise per week, along with strength training sessions.

Mix Aerobic and Strength Training

A balanced routine typically includes both aerobic (cardio) exercises and strength training. Aerobic activities improve cardiovascular health and help with weight management, while strength training enhances muscle mass and metabolism.

Start Gradually

If you're new to exercise or haven't been active for a while, start slowly and gradually increase the intensity and duration of your workouts.

Monitor Your Progress

Keep a record of your exercise sessions, noting the type, duration, and intensity. Tracking your progress can be motivating and help you make adjustments to your routine.

Vary Your Workouts

Avoid boredom and prevent overuse injuries by including a variety of exercises in your routine. Switching up activities can also work different muscle groups.

Warm-Up and Cool Down

Begin each workout with a warm-up to prepare your body and reduce the risk of injury. End with a cool-down period to gradually lower your heart rate.

Listen to Your Body

- Pay attention to how your body responds to exercise. If you experience pain or discomfort, stop and seek guidance.

Consider High-Intensity Interval Training (HIIT)

- HIIT workouts involve short bursts of intense exercise followed by brief recovery periods. HIIT can be an efficient way to improve fitness and metabolic health.

Include Flexibility and Balance

- Incorporate stretching and balance exercises, such as yoga or tai chi, into your routine to enhance overall mobility and reduce the risk of injury.

Stay Hydrated

- Drink plenty of water before, during, and after exercise to stay well-hydrated.

Make It Social

- Consider exercising with a friend or joining group fitness classes to make your workouts more enjoyable and maintain motivation.

Adjust and Progress

- As you become more fit, adjust your routine to increase intensity or challenge yourself with new exercises.

Rest and Recovery

- Allow your body time to rest and recover between intense workouts to prevent overtraining and reduce the risk of injury.

Enjoy the Outdoors

- Take advantage of outdoor activities like hiking, cycling, or jogging, which provide fresh air and a change of scenery.

Remember that consistency and finding activities you enjoy are key to a successful exercise routine. Adapt your plan as needed to ensure it remains both effective and sustainable. Consult with a fitness professional or a registered dietitian for personalized guidance and support as you work to manage insulin resistance through exercise.

Stress Management

Effective management of insulin resistance and overall health requires the management of stress. Chronic stress can hinder your body's ability to regulate blood sugar levels, which is why it is necessary to adopt stress reduction strategies. The following are some effective techniques for managing stress:

Mindfulness Meditation

Mindfulness meditation is a practice that involves focusing on the present moment and accepting it without judgment. Consistent practice can help reduce stress and improve overall well-being.

Deep Breathing Exercises

Deep breathing exercises, such as diaphragmatic breathing or the 4-7-8 technique, can help calm your nervous system and reduce stress.

Yoga

Yoga combines physical postures, breathing exercises, and relaxation techniques. It's a holistic approach to stress management that can enhance both physical and mental well-being.

Progressive Muscle Relaxation

To alleviate physical tension and stress, systematically tense and relax muscle groups with this technique.

Regular Physical Activity

Endorphins, which are natural mood lifters, are released during exercise and can help reduce stress. Incorporate regular physical activity into your routine to help manage stress.

Time Management

Effective time management can help reduce stress related to work or daily tasks. Prioritize tasks and allocate time for relaxation by creating a schedule or to-do list.

Social Support

Maintaining a strong social support network can reduce stress. Sharing your feelings and experiences with friends and family can provide emotional support.

Engage in Relaxing Hobbies

Engage in activities that you enjoy, such as reading, painting, gardening, or listening to music. Engaging in hobbies can be a form of relaxation.

Limit Caffeine and Alcohol

Excessive caffeine and alcohol intake can increase stress and anxiety. Especially in the evening, limit consumption.

Adequate Sleep

Quality sleep is essential for stress management. Establish a regular sleep schedule and create a restful sleep environment to prioritize sleep.

Seek Professional Help

Consider speaking with a mental health professional for guidance and support if stress is overwhelming and significantly affecting your daily life.

Stay Organized

Stress can be reduced and a sense of control created by staying organized and reducing clutter in your living and working spaces.

Practice Gratitude

By keeping a gratitude journal or simply reflecting on the positive aspects of your life, you can shift your focus away from stressors.

Limit Screen Time

Excessive screen time, especially before bed, can contribute to stress and sleep disturbances. Create digital-free periods in your day.

Breathing Apps and Relaxation Techniques

Guided relaxation, breathing exercises, and stress-reduction techniques are available on smartphone apps or online resources that can be utilized.

Set Boundaries

Establish clear boundaries for work and personal life to prevent overextending yourself and reduce stress from work-related pressures.

To manage insulin resistance and promote overall health, effective stress management is a valuable skill. By customizing these techniques to suit your needs and incorporating them into your daily routine, you can manage stress and promote a sense of well-being. Remember that reducing stress is an ongoing process, and it's crucial to prioritize self-care as part of your overall health strategy.

Stress levels have the potential to significantly affect blood sugar levels and insulin, which can lead to metabolic issues and insulin resistance. The following outlines how stress impacts metabolic health and insulin:

Hormones Due to Stress

When the body is under stress, it releases hormones such as cortisol and adrenaline. These hormones help to prepare the body for the "fight or flight" response, which can cause blood sugar levels to rise to provide energy for immediate action.

Increased Blood Sugar

Stress-induced hormones can cause an increase in blood sugar levels because the liver releases glucose into the bloodstream. This is a normal stress reaction, but for those with insulin resistance, it can cause prolonged and higher blood sugar elevations.

Insulin Resistance

Chronic or frequent stress can result in persistent high levels of stress hormones. Over time, this could contribute to the development of insulin resistance, making it difficult for glucose to enter cells since cells become less responsive to insulin.

Emotional Eating

Stress can trigger emotional eating, leading individuals to consume high-sugar or high-calorie foods as a coping mechanism, which can worsen blood sugar fluctuations and weight gain.

Accumulation of Abdominal Fat

Chronic stress is associated with the accumulation of abdominal fat, which is linked to an increased risk of metabolic issues and insulin resistance.

Sleep Disturbances

Stress can disrupt sleep patterns, leading to insufficient or poor-quality sleep. Inadequate sleep can negatively impact insulin sensitivity.

Unhealthy Lifestyle Choices

Under stress, individuals may be more likely to make unhealthy lifestyle choices, such as skipping exercise, smoking, or excessive alcohol consumption, which can further worsen insulin resistance and metabolic health.

Increased Inflammation

Chronic stress can lead to an increase in inflammation in the body, which is linked to insulin resistance and other metabolic issues.

Psychosocial Factors

Stress may also impact insulin resistance through psychosocial factors such as depression, anxiety, and poor adherence to medication or dietary recommendations.

It's worth noting that not all stress is harmful. Short-term stress responses can be beneficial in certain situations. However, long-term or chronic stress can lead to long-term health issues such as exacerbating insulin resistance and an increased risk of developing type 2 diabetes.

Managing stress through techniques such as mindfulness, relaxation, exercise, and social support is essential in preventing and addressing its impact on insulin and metabolic health. Additionally, seeking guidance from healthcare professionals can help you develop a personalized plan for managing stress and promoting overall well-being.

Stress Reduction Techniques

Stress management strategies can be highly effective in managing stress, improving insulin sensitivity, and promoting overall well-being. Below are some practical stress reduction techniques to consider:

Mindfulness Meditation

Mindfulness meditation involves focusing on the present moment without judgment. Regular practice can decrease stress and enhance emotional well-being.

Deep Breathing Exercises

Deep, slow breathing exercises can help soothe the nervous system and decrease stress. Experiment with techniques like diaphragmatic breathing or the 4-7-8 breath.
Progressive Muscle Relaxation

This method involves gradually tensing and relaxing muscle groups to reduce physical tension and enhance relaxation.

Yoga

Yoga blends physical postures, breathing exercises, and meditation to boost both physical and mental well-being. It's effective for decreasing stress and increasing flexibility.

Tai Chi

Tai Chi is a low-impact, mind-body exercise that emphasizes slow, flowing movements and deep breathing. It can decrease stress and improve balance.

Exercise

Regular physical activity, such as aerobic exercises and strength training, releases endorphins that act as natural mood lifters. Exercise can decrease stress and improve overall mental health.

Art and Creativity

Engaging in creative activities like art, painting, or crafting can be a form of relaxation and self-expression.

Social Support

Spending time with friends and loved ones, sharing your thoughts and feelings, and seeking support can decrease stress and provide emotional well-being.

Time Management

Effective time management can decrease stress related to work or daily tasks. Create schedules or to-do lists to prioritize tasks and allocate time for relaxation.
Adequate Sleep
- Prioritize sleep by establishing a regular sleep schedule and creating a restful sleep environment. Quality sleep is essential for stress management.

Limit Screen Time
- Reducing screen time, especially before bed, can help decrease stress and improve sleep quality.

Laughter and Humor
- Laughter is a natural stress reducer. Watch a funny movie, read a humorous book, or spend time with people who make you laugh.

Gratitude Practice
- Keeping a gratitude journal or simply reflecting on the positive aspects of your life can shift your focus away from stressors.

Relaxing Hobbies
- Pursue hobbies and activities that you enjoy, whether it's reading, gardening, or listening to music. Hobbies can be a form of relaxation.

Limit Caffeine and Alcohol
- Excessive caffeine and alcohol intake can increase stress and anxiety. Limit consumption, especially in the evening.

Seeking Professional Help
- If stress is overwhelming and significantly affecting your daily life, consider speaking with a mental health professional for guidance and support.

Nature and Outdoor Activities
- Spending time in nature, hiking, or engaging in outdoor activities can provide a sense of relaxation and connection with the natural world.

Breathing Apps and Relaxation Techniques
- Utilize smartphone apps or online resources that offer guided relaxation, breathing exercises, and stress-reduction techniques.

Customizing a combination of these stress reduction techniques to fit your preferences and needs is key to effective stress management. By prioritizing self-care and integrating these strategies into your daily routine, you can better manage stress, improve insulin sensitivity, and promote your overall health and well-being.

Practical Tips and Recipes

Of course! Here are some practical suggestions for cooking and a straightforward recipe to help you get started.

Cooking Suggestions:

Read the Recipe First before commencing cooking, read the entire recipe. This step will assist you in comprehending the process and gathering all the necessary ingredients and equipment.

Mise en Place: This French term means "everything in its place." Preparing and measuring all your ingredients before you start cooking can make the process smoother.

Knife Skills Learn basic knife skills to chop, slice, and dice ingredients quickly and safely.

Seasoning Add seasoning to your food at different stages of cooking, not just at the end. This will create layers of flavour.

Taste as You Go: Regularly taste your dish as you cook to adjust the seasoning and ensure it is turning out as expected.

Don't Overcrowd the Pan: When sautéing or stir-frying, avoid overcrowding the pan. Cook in batches if necessary to prevent food from steaming instead of browning.

Properly Cooked Meat: Purchase a meat thermometer to ensure that you cook meat to the appropriate internal temperature for safety and taste.

Clean as You Go: Keep your workspace clean by cleaning as you cook. This will make the cleanup process more manageable.

Recipe: Simple Tomato Basil Pasta

Ingredients

8 ounces of your preferred pasta (e.g., spaghetti, penne)
2 tablespoons of olive oil
3 cloves of garlic, minced
1 can (14 oz) of crushed tomatoes
Salt and pepper to taste
1/2 teaspoon of red pepper flakes (adjust to your spice preference)
1/2 cup of fresh basil leaves, torn or chopped
Grated Parmesan cheese (optional)

Instructions

Cook the pasta Bring a large pot of salted
water to a boil. Add the pasta and cook
according to the package instructions until the
pasta is al dente. Drain the pasta and set it
aside.

Make the sauce In a large skillet, heat the olive
oil over medium heat. Add the minced garlic
and red pepper flakes. Sauté for about 1-2
minutes or until the garlic becomes fragrant.

Add the crushed tomatoes to the skillet. Season
with salt and pepper to taste. Simmer the sauce
for about 10-15 minutes, stirring occasionally,
until it thickens.

Stir in the torn or chopped fresh basil and let it
cook for an additional 2-3 minutes.

Combine the cooked pasta and the tomato basil
sauce in the skillet. Toss to coat the pasta
evenly with the sauce.

Serve hot, garnished with grated Parmesan
cheese if desired.

This simple and delicious tomato basil pasta is
a quick and satisfying meal that you can
prepare with ease. Enjoy your homemade dish!

Eating Out with Insulin Resistance

When dining out with insulin resistance, it's essential to make mindful choices to manage blood sugar levels effectively. Here are some tips:

Choose Complex Carbs Opt for whole grains like brown rice, quinoa, or whole wheat instead of refined carbohydrates. These complex carbs have a slower impact on blood sugar.

Lean Proteins Include lean proteins such as grilled chicken, fish, or tofu in your meal. Protein helps stabilize blood sugar levels and keeps you feeling full.

Healthy Fats Incorporate sources of healthy fats, like avocados, nuts, and olive oil. These fats can slow down the digestion of carbohydrates, preventing rapid spikes in blood sugar.

Portion Control Be mindful of portion sizes. Consider sharing a dish or asking for a smaller portion to avoid overeating.

Fiber-Rich Choices Foods high in fiber, such as vegetables and legumes, can help regulate blood sugar. Include a variety of colorful vegetables in your meal.

Limit Sugary Drinks Opt for water, herbal tea, or drinks without added sugars. Sugary beverages can lead to rapid increases in blood sugar.

Choose Grilled or Baked Options Select grilled, baked, or steamed dishes instead of fried options. This reduces the intake of unhealthy fats.

Watch for Hidden Sugars Be aware of sauces, dressings, and marinades that may contain hidden sugars. Ask for them on the side to control the amount you consume.

Mindful Eating Eat slowly and savor each bite. This gives your body time to recognize signals of fullness, preventing overeating.

Inform Restaurant Staff If you have specific dietary needs or restrictions, don't hesitate to inform the restaurant staff. Many places can accommodate special requests.

Remember to listen to your body and monitor how different foods affect your blood sugar levels. Making informed choices while dining out can help you enjoy meals without compromising your health.

Making Smart Choices at Restaurants

Certainly! Making smart choices at restaurants is crucial when managing insulin levels. Here are some tips to help you make informed decisions:

Review the Menu in Advance: Many restaurants provide their menus online. Take the time to review the options beforehand, so you can plan a balanced meal.

Choose Lean Proteins Opt for lean protein sources like grilled chicken, fish, or tofu. Protein helps stabilize blood sugar levels and keeps you feeling full.

Select Whole Grains:Choose whole grains over refined carbohydrates. Options like brown rice, quinoa, or whole wheat pasta have a lower impact on blood sugar.

Load Up on Vegetables incorporate a variety of vegetables into your meal. They are rich in fiber and essential nutrients while being lower in carbohydrates.

Watch Portion Sizes be mindful of portion sizes. Consider sharing an entree or ask for a smaller portion to avoid overeating.

Ask for Modifications Don't hesitate to ask for modifications to suit your dietary needs. For example, request grilled instead of fried, or ask for sauces and dressings on the side.

Be Wary of Sugary Sauces Watch out for sauces and condiments that may contain added sugars. Choose options with minimal or no sugar, and use them sparingly.

Avoid Sugary Beverages opt for water, unsweetened tea, or other low-calorie beverages instead of sugary drinks. This helps control your overall carbohydrate intake.

Limit Alcoholic Beverages If you choose to have alcohol, do so in moderation. Alcoholic drinks can affect blood sugar levels, so monitor your intake and choose lower-carb options.

Skip the Dessert or Share Desserts are often high in sugars and carbohydrates. Consider skipping dessert or sharing it with others to manage your carb intake.

Monitor Blood Sugar Levels Regularly monitor your blood sugar levels, especially if you're trying new foods. This can help you understand how different choices impact your body.

Plan for Physical Activity If possible, plan some physical activity after your meal. This can help regulate blood sugar levels and improve insulin sensitivity.

Remember, making smart choices at restaurants is about balance and awareness. By being proactive and informed, you can enjoy dining out while managing your insulin levels effectively.

Absolutely! Here are two delicious and nutritious recipes to try

Grilled Salmon with Quinoa and Roasted Vegetables.

Ingredients

2 salmon filets
1 cup quinoa, rinsed
2 cups mixed vegetables (e.g., bell peppers, zucchini, cherry tomatoes)
2 tablespoons olive oil
2 cloves garlic, minced
1 teaspoon dried oregano
Salt and pepper to taste
Lemon wedges for garnish

Instructions

Preheat the grill or oven to medium-high heat.

Season the salmon filets with salt.

Breakfast Options

Certainly! Here are two breakfast options that are balanced and suitable for managing insulin levels

Greek Yogurt Parfait

Ingredients

1 cup Greek yogurt (unsweetened)
1/2 cup mixed berries (e.g., blueberries, strawberries)
1/4 cup granola (choose a variety with low added sugars)
1 tablespoon chia seeds
1 drizzle of honey (optional)

Instructions

In a bowl or glass, layer Greek yoghurt at the bottom.

Add a layer of mixed berries on top of the yoghurt.

Sprinkle granola over the berries.

Add chia seeds for an extra boost of fiber.

Optionally, drizzle a small amount of honey for sweetness.

Repeat the layers if desired.

Enjoy a delicious and nutrient-packed Greek yoghurt parfait.

2. Veggie Omelette with Whole Grain Toast:

Ingredients

2 eggs
1/4 cup diced bell peppers (mixed colours)
1/4 cup diced tomatoes
1/4 cup chopped spinach
1/4 cup shredded mozzarella cheese
Salt and pepper to taste
1 teaspoon olive oil
1 slice whole grain bread

Instructions

In a bowl, beat the eggs and season with salt and pepper.

Heat olive oil in a non-stick skillet over medium heat.

Add diced bell peppers, tomatoes, and chopped spinach to the skillet. Sauté until vegetables are tender.

Pour the beaten eggs over the vegetables in the skillet.

Once the edges start to set, lift them with a spatula to let the uncooked eggs flow underneath.

Sprinkle shredded mozzarella cheese over one-half of the omelet.

Fold the omelet in half and cook until the cheese is melted and the eggs are fully cooked.

Toast a slice of whole-grain bread.

Serve the omelet with the whole grain toast on the side.

These breakfast options provide a good balance of protein, healthy fats, and complex carbohydrates, helping to manage insulin levels effectively. Adjust portion sizes based on individual dietary needs and preferences.

Of course! Here are two recipes for lunch and dinner that are well-balanced and can help manage insulin levels:

Grilled Chicken Salad

Ingredients

- 4 oz grilled chicken breast, sliced
- 2 cups mixed salad greens (such as spinach, arugula, or romaine)
- 1/2 cup halved cherry tomatoes
- 1/4 sliced cucumber
- 1/4 sliced red bell pepper
- 1/4 cup crumbled feta cheese
- 1 tbsp olive oil
- 1 tbsp balsamic vinegar
- Salt and pepper to taste
- 1 tbsp sunflower seeds (optional)

Instructions

- Season the grilled chicken with salt and pepper, then slice it into strips.
- In a large bowl, combine the mixed salad greens, cherry tomatoes, cucumber, red bell pepper, and grilled chicken.
- In a small bowl, whisk together the olive oil and balsamic vinegar, then drizzle the dressing over the salad and toss to combine.
- Sprinkle crumbled feta cheese and sunflower seeds over the salad.
- Serve immediately for a satisfying and refreshing grilled chicken salad.

Baked Salmon with Quinoa and Steamed Vegetables

Ingredients

- 2 salmon fillets
- 1 cup rinsed quinoa
- 2 cups broccoli florets
- 1 thinly sliced carrot
- 1 tbsp olive oil
- 1 sliced lemon
- 2 tbsp chopped fresh dill
- Salt and pepper to taste

Instructions

- Preheat the oven to 375°F (190°C).
- Place the salmon fillets on a baking sheet lined with parchment paper. Season with salt and pepper, then top with lemon slices and chopped dill.
- Bake the salmon in the preheated oven for 15-20 minutes or until it flakes easily with a fork.
- In a saucepan, bring 2 cups of water to a boil, then add quinoa. Reduce heat to low, cover, and simmer for 15 minutes or until the quinoa is cooked.
- While the salmon is baking and quinoa is cooking, steam the broccoli and carrot until they are tender-crisp.
- Drizzle olive oil over the steamed vegetables and season with salt and pepper.
- Serve the baked salmon over a bed of cooked quinoa, accompanied by the steamed vegetables.

These recipes include lean proteins, whole grains, and an abundance of vegetables, which can provide a nutritious and well-balanced option for both lunch and dinner while also supporting insulin management. Adjust portion sizes as needed. Enjoy your delicious and healthy meals!

Sure, I can help you with that. Here are three snack options that are mindful of insulin management:

Greek Yogurt and Berry Parfait

Ingredients

- 1/2 cup of unsweetened Greek yogurt
- 1/2 cup of mixed berries (such as blueberries and raspberries)
- 1 tablespoon of chia seeds
- 1 tablespoon of chopped nuts (such as almonds and walnuts)
- Optional: a drizzle of honey

Instructions

- Add a layer of Greek yogurt to a bowl or glass.
- Top the yogurt with a layer of mixed berries.
- Sprinkle chia seeds and chopped nuts over the berries.
- For sweetness, you can add a small amount of honey, if desired.
- Stir gently and enjoy a delicious and protein-rich Greek yogurt parfait.

Veggie Sticks with Hummus

Ingredients

- 1 cup of baby carrots and cucumber sticks
- 2 tablespoons of hummus (choose a variety without added sugars)
- Cherry tomatoes for extra color

Instructions

- Arrange baby carrots, cucumber sticks, and cherry tomatoes on a plate.
- Serve with a side of hummus for dipping.
- Enjoy a crunchy and satisfying snack that combines fiber, healthy fats, and protein.

Baked Apple Slices with Cinnamon

Ingredients

- 1 sliced and cored apple
- 1/2 teaspoon of cinnamon
- 1 tablespoon of chopped nuts (such as walnuts and almonds)

Instructions

- Preheat your oven to 350°F (175°C).
- Place the apple slices on a baking sheet lined with parchment paper.
- Sprinkle cinnamon over the apple slices.
- Bake in the preheated oven for 15-20 minutes or until the apples are tender.
- Sprinkle the chopped nuts over the baked apple slices before serving.
- Enjoy a warm and comforting dessert that is low in added sugars.

These snack and dessert options feature whole foods, include fiber, healthy fats, and protein, and can help manage insulin levels effectively. Remember to adjust portion sizes based on individual dietary needs and preferences.

Monitoring and tracking your progress is crucial when managing insulin levels. Here are key aspects to consider:

Blood Glucose Monitoring

Regularly check your blood glucose levels as recommended by your healthcare provider. This helps you understand how your body responds to different foods, activities, and medications.

Food Journaling

Keep a detailed food journal to track your meals, snacks, and portion sizes. This can help identify patterns and correlations between your food choices and blood sugar levels.

Carbohydrate Counting

Learn to count carbohydrates in your meals. This empowers you to make informed decisions about your food intake and helps maintain more stable blood sugar levels.

Physical Activity Log

Record your physical activity, including the type, duration, and intensity. Regular exercise can improve insulin sensitivity and contribute to better blood sugar control.

Medication Adherence

If you are prescribed insulin or other medications, adhere to your medication schedule. Keep track of any changes in dosage or timing under the guidance of your healthcare team.
Regular Healthcare Checkups

Schedule regular checkups with your healthcare provider to discuss your progress. They can adjust your treatment plan based on your evolving needs and provide valuable insights.

Symptom Monitoring

Be mindful of any changes in symptoms related to insulin resistance, such as increased thirst, frequent urination, or fatigue. Report these changes to your healthcare provider promptly.
Lifestyle Modifications

Evaluate lifestyle factors, including stress levels and sleep patterns. Stress management and adequate sleep contribute to overall well-being and can impact insulin sensitivity.

Set Realistic Goals

Establish realistic and achievable goals for your insulin management. These could include reaching and maintaining a target blood sugar level, losing weight if necessary, or adopting a more active lifestyle.

Educational Resources

Stay informed about insulin resistance and diabetes management through reputable sources. Education empowers you to make informed decisions about your health.

Celebrate Successes

Celebrate your achievements, no matter how small. Recognizing your progress can be motivating and reinforce positive behaviors.

Consult with the Healthcare Team

Work closely with your healthcare team, including your doctor, dietitian, and diabetes educator. They can provide personalized guidance based on your individual needs. Remember, managing insulin levels is a dynamic process, and what works for one person may vary for another. Regular monitoring, coupled with a holistic approach to health, can contribute to better insulin control and an improved overall quality of life.

Tracking Your Progress

Certainly! Tracking your progress in managing insulin involves a holistic approach that extends beyond numerical values. Here's more on this crucial aspect:

Mindful Eating Practices

Pay attention to how you eat, not just what you eat. Mindful eating involves savouring each bite, recognizing hunger and fullness cues, and appreciating the sensory experience of your meals.

Hydration Habits

Monitor your water intake. Staying adequately hydrated supports overall health and can positively influence blood sugar levels. Aim for consistent hydration throughout the day.

Stress Management

Keep tabs on stress levels. Chronic stress can impact insulin resistance. Incorporate stress-relieving activities into your routine, such as deep breathing, meditation, or hobbies that bring joy.

Sleep Quality

Track your sleep patterns. Aim for a consistent sleep schedule and prioritize quality sleep. Poor sleep can affect insulin sensitivity and overall well-being.
Physical Fitness Progress:

Evaluate changes in your fitness routine. As you engage in regular physical activity, note improvements in stamina, strength, or flexibility. Adjust your exercise regimen based on your evolving fitness goals.

Medication Adjustments

Document any medication adjustments. If your healthcare provider modifies your treatment plan, monitor how these changes impact your blood sugar levels and overall health.

Lifestyle Modifications

Keep a log of lifestyle changes. Whether it's incorporating more vegetables into your diet, reducing processed foods, or taking the stairs instead of the elevator, document positive lifestyle modifications.

Blood Pressure and Cholesterol Levels

Include regular checks of blood pressure and cholesterol levels in your tracking routine. These factors are interconnected with insulin resistance and contribute to your overall cardiovascular health.

Emotional Well-being

Assess your emotional well-being. A positive mindset and emotional resilience can positively influence your ability to manage insulin levels. Seek support from friends, family, or professionals if needed.

Education and Empowerment

Keep learning about insulin resistance and diabetes management. Stay informed about new research, technologies, and lifestyle strategies. Knowledge empowers you to make informed decisions about your health.

Celebrate Non-Scale Victories

Acknowledge and celebrate non-scale victories. Whether it's consistently choosing nutritious foods, maintaining a regular exercise routine, or practicing self-care, recognize these achievements on your journey.
Remember, tracking progress is not only about numbers but also about the positive changes you incorporate into your daily life. By paying attention to various aspects of your well-being, you create a comprehensive approach to managing insulin levels effectively.

Keeping a Food Diary

It can be helpful for individuals who are managing their insulin levels to maintain a food diary. The following are reasons why and suggestions on how to maintain an effective food diary:

Importance of Keeping a Food Diary

Insight into Eating Patterns:

By keeping track of your daily food intake, a food diary can help you identify trends and patterns in your eating habits. This information is crucial for understanding how different foods affect your blood sugar levels.

Carbohydrate Tracking

Tracking the types and amounts of carbohydrates you consume is beneficial for managing insulin dosage. This awareness enables you to make informed decisions about the composition of your meals.

Identification of Trigger Foods

A food diary can help you pinpoint specific foods that may cause spikes or drops in blood sugar levels. Identifying these trigger foods allows you to make strategic adjustments to your diet.

Portion Control

Monitoring portion sizes is important for maintaining consistent blood sugar levels. A food diary helps you determine appropriate serving sizes, preventing overconsumption of carbohydrates.

Meal Timing

Keeping track of when you eat can reveal patterns related to blood sugar fluctuations.

Understanding the timing of meals allows for better coordination between insulin administration and food intake.

Behavioural Insights

Keeping track of emotional or stress-related eating can provide insights into how emotions influence dietary choices. This awareness helps in developing strategies to manage stress without relying on unhealthy food choices.

Tips for Keeping an Effective Food Diary

Be Detailed

Record everything you eat and drink, including snacks and beverages. Note portion sizes, cooking methods, and any condiments used. Include Blood Sugar Readings

Pair food entries with blood sugar readings to establish connections between your dietary choices and their impact on glucose levels. Record Meal Times

Note the times at which you consume meals and snacks. This helps in creating a consistent

eating schedule, which is beneficial for insulin management.
Describe Feelings and Context:

Include notes on your emotional state and any environmental factors during meals. This provides a comprehensive view of the circumstances surrounding your eating habits.
Use Apps or Templates

Explore food diary apps or templates that make the tracking process more convenient. These tools often calculate nutritional information and may provide insights into dietary patterns.
Review Regularly

Set aside time to review your food diary regularly. Look for trends, identify potential areas for improvement, and celebrate positive dietary choices.
Share with Healthcare Provider

Share your food diary with your healthcare provider. This collaboration allows them to tailor insulin management strategies based on your specific dietary patterns and needs. Maintaining a food diary is a proactive step towards achieving better control over insulin levels. It serves as a personal guide, offering valuable information for informed decision-making and creating a more personalized approach to insulin management.

Regular Check-Ins

Regular check-ins for insulin management are crucial to ensure effective control of blood sugar levels. Here's why and how to conduct these check-ins:

Importance of Regular Check-Ins

Monitoring Blood Sugar Levels

Regular check-ins involve monitoring your blood sugar levels consistently. This helps you understand how well your current insulin regimen is working and allows for timely adjustments.

Assessing Insulin Sensitivity

Monitoring trends in blood sugar readings helps assess your body's sensitivity to insulin. Recognizing patterns allows for fine-tuning insulin doses based on specific needs.

Detecting Changes in Lifestyle or Diet

Regular check-ins help identify changes in lifestyle, diet, or activity levels that may impact insulin requirements. Adjusting insulin accordingly ensures it aligns with your current habits.

Preventing Hypoglycemia or Hyperglycemia

Monitoring blood sugar levels prevents extremes—both hypoglycemia (low blood sugar) and hyperglycemia (high blood sugar). Timely interventions can help avoid complications associated with these conditions.

Evaluating Medication Adherence

Regular check-ins provide an opportunity to discuss medication adherence. Confirming that insulin is taken as prescribed ensures its effectiveness in managing blood sugar levels.

Assessing Overall Health

Checking in regularly allows healthcare providers to assess your overall health. They can address any concerns, monitor for potential complications, and guide on maintaining a healthy lifestyle.

How to Conduct Regular Check-Ins

Schedule Appointments

Schedule regular appointments with your healthcare provider for comprehensive check-ins. The frequency of these appointments may vary based on individual needs and healthcare recommendations.

Blood Sugar Monitoring

Monitor your blood sugar levels as recommended by your healthcare team. Regularly checking at home provides valuable data for discussions during check-ins.

Communication with Healthcare Providers

Communicate openly with your healthcare provider about any changes in lifestyle, diet, or physical activity. Share concerns or challenges you may be facing in managing insulin effectively.

Reviewing Trends

Review trends in blood sugar readings with your healthcare team. Identify any consistent patterns or irregularities that may require adjustments in your insulin regimen.

Medication Adjustments

Based on discussions and blood sugar trends, your healthcare provider may suggest adjustments to your insulin dosage or timing. Adhere to any changes recommended during these check-ins.

Discussing Challenges

Use check-ins to discuss any challenges you face in managing insulin. This could include issues with injection sites, side effects, or difficulties in adhering to the prescribed regimen.

Setting Goals

Collaborate with your healthcare provider to set realistic and achievable goals for insulin management. These goals could focus on maintaining target blood sugar levels, improving lifestyle factors, or addressing specific concerns.

Regular check-ins ensure a proactive and collaborative approach to managing insulin. They provide an opportunity to address challenges, make informed adjustments, and work towards achieving optimal blood sugar control for improved overall health.

Conclusion

In conclusion, managing insulin effectively is a dynamic and personalized journey that requires continuous attention and collaboration. By incorporating mindful practices such as regular blood sugar monitoring, maintaining a detailed food diary, and engaging in regular check-ins with healthcare providers, individuals can navigate the intricacies of insulin management with greater success.

It's essential to view insulin management not just as a medical regimen but as an integral part of a holistic approach to health. Lifestyle factors, including nutrition, physical activity, stress management, and sleep quality, play pivotal roles in achieving optimal blood sugar control.

Moreover, tracking progress extends beyond numerical values to encompass positive changes in behaviour, emotional well-being, and overall lifestyle choices. Celebrating non-scale victories and acknowledging the efforts put into maintaining a healthy balance contribute significantly to the overall success of insulin management.

Education and empowerment remain key components of this journey. Staying informed about insulin resistance, diabetes management, and emerging research allows individuals to make informed decisions, adapt to new strategies, and actively participate in their healthcare.

In the broader context, the journey of insulin management is not isolated but rather interconnected with the individual's unique life circumstances. Regular reflection, adjustment, and the incorporation of lessons learned contribute to ongoing success in maintaining stable blood sugar levels.

In embracing this holistic perspective, individuals can approach insulin management with resilience, understanding that it's not just about managing a medical condition but cultivating a lifestyle that fosters long-term well-being. Ultimately, the journey with insulin is a partnership—between individuals, their healthcare providers, and the choices they make each day in pursuit of a healthier and more fulfilling life.

The Road to Better Health

The road to better health is a transformative journey that involves conscious choices, commitment, and a holistic approach to well-being. Here are key elements to consider on this empowering path.

Nutritious Eating

Choose whole, nutrient-dense foods that nourish your body. Prioritize a balanced intake of lean proteins, colourful vegetables, whole grains, and healthy fats. Be mindful of portion sizes and stay hydrated.

Regular Physical Activity

Incorporate regular exercise into your routine. Whether it's walking, jogging, dancing, or engaging in a favourite sport, physical activity not only supports weight management but also boosts mood and enhances overall health.

Mindful Stress Management

Develop effective stress management strategies. Incorporate practices such as meditation, deep breathing, or yoga to reduce stress levels. Recognize the importance of mental well-being in achieving holistic health.

Adequate Sleep

Prioritize quality sleep for optimal health. Create a sleep-friendly environment, maintain a consistent sleep schedule, and ensure you get the recommended amount of rest each night. Quality sleep contributes to physical and mental resilience.

Hydration Habits

Stay adequately hydrated throughout the day. Water is essential for numerous bodily functions, including digestion, metabolism, and detoxification. Limit sugary beverages and prioritize water as your primary source of hydration.

Regular Health Check-Ups

Schedule routine check-ups with your healthcare provider. Regular health assessments and screenings allow for early detection of potential issues and provide a baseline for tracking overall health progress.

Healthy Lifestyle Choices

Make conscious lifestyle choices that align with your well-being goals. This includes avoiding smoking, limiting alcohol intake, and minimizing exposure to environmental toxins. Small, positive changes can have a significant impact on long-term health.

Continuous Learning and Adaptation

Stay informed about health-related topics. Continuous learning empowers you to make informed decisions, adapt to new information, and take an active role in your health journey. Seek reliable sources for information and consult healthcare professionals when needed.

Cultivating Positive Relationships

Nurture positive relationships with friends, family, and your community. Social connections contribute to emotional well-being and provide support during challenging times. Surround yourself with a supportive network.

Mental and Emotional Well-being

- Prioritize mental and emotional health.
Practice self-care, engage in activities you
enjoy, and seek professional support if needed.
Emotional well-being is integral to achieving a
balanced and fulfilling life.

Remember, the road to better health is a
continuous, dynamic journey. It's not about
perfection but about making consistent,
positive choices that align with your individual
needs and goals. Celebrate the progress you
make along the way, embrace the lessons
learned, and cultivate a lifestyle that fosters a
healthier and more vibrant you.

Resources and Further Reading

Certainly! Here are some valuable resources and suggested readings to enhance your understanding of insulin management, diabetes, and overall health:

Books

"Think Like a Pancreas: A Practical Guide to Managing Diabetes with Insulin" by Gary Scheiner

This book provides practical insights and strategies for effectively managing diabetes with a focus on insulin therapy.
"The Blood Sugar Solution: The UltraHealthy Program for Losing Weight, Preventing Disease, and Feeling Great Now!" by Mark Hyman

Dr. Mark Hyman offers a comprehensive guide that addresses the root causes of insulin resistance and provides actionable steps for achieving optimal health.
"The Diabetes Code: Prevent and Reverse Type 2 Diabetes Naturally" by Jason Fung

Dr. Jason Fung explores the role of insulin in diabetes and provides insights into preventing and reversing type 2 diabetes through lifestyle changes.
Websites and Online Resources:

American Diabetes Association (ADA)

Website: American Diabetes Association
The ADA offers a wealth of information on diabetes, insulin management, and healthy living.
National Institute of Diabetes and Digestive and Kidney Diseases (NIDDK):

Website: NIDDK
NIDDK provides resources and research updates on diabetes and related conditions.
Diabetes Forecast:

Website: Diabetes Forecast
Diabetes Forecast, the consumer magazine of the ADA, offers articles, recipes, and lifestyle tips for people with diabetes.

Apps

mySugr: Diabetes Tracker Log

An app designed to help you log and monitor blood sugar levels, meals, and other aspects of diabetes management.
Carb Manager: Keto Diet App

While originally focused on low-carb diets, Carb Manager can be useful for tracking carb intake and nutritional information.

Podcasts

The Diabetes Connection Podcast

Hosted by Stacey Simms, this podcast covers a variety of topics related to diabetes management, including insulin use and technological advancements.

Mastering Diabetes Podcast

Co-hosted by Cyrus Khambatta, PhD, and Robby Barbaro, MPH, this podcast explores plant-based nutrition and its impact on diabetes management.

These resources offer a combination of practical advice, expert insights, and community support to assist you in your journey towards better insulin management and overall health. Always consult with your healthcare provider for personalized guidance based on your individual needs and circumstances.

Appendix Vs Glossary of Terms

Certainly! Let's distinguish between an appendix and a glossary of terms

Appendix

An appendix is a supplementary section at the end of a document, often used to provide additional information that is not essential to the main content but supports and enhances understanding.
It typically includes detailed data, technical information, charts, graphs, or lengthy explanations that would disrupt the flow of the main text if included within it.
Appendices are labeled numerically or alphabetically (e.g., Appendix A, Appendix B) and are referenced in the main text.

Glossary of Terms

A glossary is a section within a document that defines and explains specialized or unfamiliar terms used in the content.
It serves to clarify the meanings of words or phrases that might be unclear to the reader,

providing a quick reference for understanding key terminology.

Glossary entries are usually listed alphabetically and include the term's definition or explanation.

Key Differences

An appendix provides supplementary material, while a glossary focuses on defining terms.

Appendices are typically located at the end of a document, whereas a glossary can be placed at the end or within the document, depending on the author's preference.

Appendices may include various types of content, such as tables, figures, or extended explanations, while a glossary is specifically dedicated to defining terms.

In summary, an appendix is a section for additional content, while a glossary is a section for defining terms, both serving to enhance the reader's understanding of the document.

Certainly! When managing insulin resistance, focusing on a balanced and nutrient-dense diet is key. Here are some insulin-resistance-friendly food lists to guide your food choices:

Non-Starchy Vegetables:l

Leafy greens (spinach, kale, arugula)
Cruciferous vegetables (broccoli, cauliflower, Brussels sprouts)
Bell peppers
Cucumber
Zucchini
Asparagus

Lean Proteins

Chicken breast
Turkey
Fish (salmon, trout, tuna)
Eggs
Greek yogurt (unsweetened)
Tofu or tempeh

Whole Grains and Complex Carbohydrates

Quinoa
Brown rice
Oats (steel-cut or old-fashioned)
Barley
Sweet potatoes
Legumes (lentils, chickpeas, black beans)

Healthy Fats

Avocado
Olive oil
Nuts (almonds, walnuts, pistachios)
Seeds (flaxseeds, chia seeds)
Fatty fish (salmon, mackerel)

Low-Glycemic Fruits

Berries (blueberries, strawberries, raspberries)
Cherries
Apples
Pears
Plums
Peaches

Dairy or Dairy Alternatives

Greek yogurt (unsweetened)
Cottage cheese
Almond milk or coconut milk (unsweetened)

Herbs and Spices

Cinnamon
Turmeric
Garlic
Ginger
Basil
Cilantro

Beverages

Water
Herbal teas (unsweetened)
Green tea

Foods to Limit or Avoid

Refined sugars and sweets
Processed and packaged foods
White bread and refined grains
Sweetened beverages
High-sugar fruits in excess (grapes,
watermelon)

Remember, these lists are general guidelines and individual responses to foods may vary. It's essential to monitor blood sugar levels and work with healthcare professionals to create a personalized meal plan that suits your specific needs and preferences. Additionally, focusing on portion control and spreading meals throughout the day can help manage insulin resistance more effectively.

This comprehensive table of contents will guide readers through, managing, and improving their insulin resistance through dietary and lifestyle changes.